'This volume is a must have for affirmatively working with queer clients and their relationships of today and tomorrow. *Relationally Queer* is as ground breaking to the psychotherapy field as earlier volumes of the Pink Therapy series. Chapters address areas ranging from challenging monogamy to counselling people who sex work to addressing health issues – and more! A thoughtful overview of the gender, sex, and relationship diversities (GSRD) framework is also provided'.

Markie L.C Twist, PHD, LMFT, LMHC, CSE-S,
Teaching Faculty, Antioch University New England;
Editor-in-Chief, Sexual and Relationship Therapy

'Having trained relationship therapists – globally – for decades GSRD is of great value to me: it recognises, defines and positions a wide range of relationship expressions as either including **everyone** (and especially indigenous groups) or to stand accused of perpetuating colonialism. This work hits the spot and I commend the authors for this ground-breaking, courageous work. I am particularly excited by the chapters on collectivist communities (African, Jewish, Muslim et al) in which individualist psychotherapy models have limited value'.

Bernd Leygraf, *Consultant Psychotherapist, CEO Naos-Institute*
(www.naos-institute.com and www.psychosexualtraining.org.uk)

'*Relationally Queer* is THE book that all GSRD specialists (including mental health professionals in training) are waiting for. The publication fills in the gaps in existing writings on the topic. It not only gives a fresh perspective of how to talk about and talk to GSRD clients but also how to include practical tools into the therapeutical space. The importance of perspective "nothing about us without us" can help us create safer environment and change the world'.

Agata Loewe-Kurilla, PhD, *Psychotherapist, Sexologist,*
Sexospher and Tutor. Founder of Sex Positive Institute

Relationally Queer

Relationally Queer explores diverse intimate relationship styles and the connections with self for clinicians interested in gender, sex and relationship diversity.

Offering readers a more inclusive and queer-friendly way of thinking about relationships, the book covers a range of topics that include intersectionality, consensual non-monogamy, working with shame, intimate partner violence, religious identities and living with HIV. Exploring beyond a Eurocentric perspective, the book features a chapter on African-centred therapy and also includes the relationships of often erased populations such as bisexual people, sex workers, people with chronic health issues and trans people.

The book will help psychosexual and relationship therapists, counsellors and psychologists who work with clients of diverse genders, sexualities and relationships.

Silva Neves is a COSRT-accredited and UKCP-registered psychotherapist specialising in sexology and intimate relationships. He is a Pink Therapy clinical associate. He is a course director for the Contemporary Institute of Clinical Sexology (CICS), an international speaker, broadcaster and author.

Dominic Davies is the Founder of Pink Therapy, a clinical supervisor and sexologist and course director of two training programmes in gender, sex and relationship diversity therapy. He has been internationally recognised as one of 50 gender and sexual health revolutionaries.

Relationally Queer

A Pink Therapy Guide for Practitioners

Edited by Silva Neves and Dominic Davies

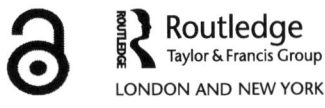

Routledge
Taylor & Francis Group
LONDON AND NEW YORK

Designed cover image: © Thomas Dyson

First published 2023
by Routledge
4 Park Square, Milton Park, Abingdon, Oxon OX14 4RN

and by Routledge
605 Third Avenue, New York, NY 10158

Routledge is an imprint of the Taylor & Francis Group, an informa business

British Library Cataloguing-in-Publication Data
A catalogue record for this book is available from the British Library

ISBN: 978-1-032-19725-8 (hbk)
ISBN: 978-1-032-19724-1 (pbk)
ISBN: 978-1-003-26056-1 (ebk)

DOI: 10.4324/9781003260561

The Open Access version of chapter 1 was funded by Y. Gávriel Ansara.

Contents

Acknowledgements

Silva and Dominic would like to thank:

All our authors who contributed chapters for this book. We are grateful for their hard work, their time and for sharing their expert knowledge.

Our dear colleague Meg-John Barker for writing a Foreword to the book and offering excellent coaching to some of our authors who were writing for print for the first time.

Dr Agata Loewe-Kurilla, Professor Markie L.C Twist and Bernd Leygraf for being willing to read a draft of the book and say great things about it on the back cover.

Thanks, too, to Thomas Dyson for the fab book cover.

We would also like to thank the people of Pignetto in Rome, the neighbourhood where we completed this book. To Nadia, our Airbnb host, the cafe owners, restauranteurs and gelateria all contributed vital sustenance in our short breaks away from the laptops.

We are both sustained by the 3,000 therapists on our Pink Therapy Facebook group and supported by the volunteer moderators. We are incredibly grateful to our students, who entrust us with their hearts and minds to train them to serve our GSRD communities better.

Silva would like to thank:

Dominic Davies for being a wonderful co-editor on this book and being so generous with his knowledge and great clinical experience.

My colleagues and friends whose love, kindness and support are invaluable: Julie Sale, Rima Hawkins, Lorraine McGinlay, Dr Francesca Tripoli, Babette Rothschild, Kate Moyle, Dr Roberta Babb, Lohani Noor, Aoife Drury, Remziye Kunelaki, Juliette Clancy, Lisa Etherson, Diana Moffat, Andrew Mirrlees, Julie Gaudion, David Piner and Clare Staunton, to name just a few. I'm so lucky to have them in my life.

My followers on my professional social media platforms who identify as Queer and Queer allies. It feels good to see them out there.

The College of Sexual and Relationship Therapists (COSRT). I'm proud to be an accredited member.

My husband, Dr James Rafferty, for his consistent love and unwavering support of my work. He brings much Queer joy to my life.

Dominic would like to thank:

Silva Neves for inviting me to be a part of this project and making the work tremendous fun.

Antonio Prunas, Maria Kindstedt and Agata Loewe-Kurilla for their constructive feedback on my chapter: your collective wisdom was invaluable, and I appreciate your intelligence, friendship and collegiality.

I am also sustained within Pink Therapy by a small and vital team of colleagues undertaking various admin roles that are necessary but distract me from focussing on the bigger picture. Thank you: Anya, Jo, Henry and Tom.

Last but not least, My partner Dodain has always been incredibly supportive and understanding of my passion for my work and time away from teaching and writing. Your love, kindness and generosity are always infallible.

Contributors

Saquib Ahmad is Consultant Psychotherapist and Activist, consulting for LGBTI NGOs internationally. He is accredited in CBT and EMDR and is a Supervisor and Trainer with specialisms in working with GSRD and trauma clients. His 'Gay Boys To Men' project has worked with over 700+ gay, bi and trans men world-wide.

Dr Y Gávriel Ansara (he/him) lives on unceded Boonwurrung Country. He is a polycultural psychotherapist, educator and supervisor specialising in anti-oppressive/liberating practice approaches. He has received awards for his research, teaching and international human rights and social justice contributions. His positioning statement on his lived experiences of oppression and privilege is available at https://liberatingcentre.care/gavi/

Dr Daniel Bąk, PhD – EAGT-accredited Gestalt Psychotherapist, also Supervisor, and Psychotherapy Teacher. He specialises in GSRD-affirmative work. A clinical associate and faculty member in Pink Therapy, UK, Bąk is also a member of the Research Council at the Centre for Social Queer Studies, University of Warsaw. He lives and works in Warsaw, Poland.

Dr Meg-John Barker is the author of several popular books on sex, gender, relationships and mental health, including graphic guides to *Queer, Gender*, and *Sexuality* (with Jules Scheele), *How To Understand Your Gender*, and *Sexuality*, *Life Isn't Binary*, and *Hell Yeah Self-Care* (with Alex Iantaffi), *Enjoy Sex* (with Justin Hancock), and *Rewriting the Rules*. They have also written a number of books and articles for scholars and counsellors on these themes, drawing on their own years of academic work and therapeutic practice, including the BACP resource on GSRD. Website: rewriting-the-rules.com.

Niki D is an existential psychotherapist with 30 years of experience in private practice, statutory and voluntary sectors. She works as a relationship therapist and holds therapy groups for therapists and GSRD people. Niki is a supervisor, clinical associate of Pink Therapy, and a visiting lecturer at Regents University, London.

Cyndi Darnell is an Australian sexologist based in NYC. Informed by feminist, sex-worker affirming, anti-racist, narrative and somatic frameworks, her previous clinical publications cover using porn within therapy, sexological group work, somatics within sex therapy and critiquing consent culture. In 2022 she published *Sex When You Don't Feel Like It* (Rowman & Littlefield).

Dr Susannah Grant is a HCPC practitioner psychologist, BPS chartered counselling psychologist, and relationship therapist. Susannah has been working in the field of adult mental health since 2009. She currently works in private practice in the UK, where she sees clients from the LGBTQIA+ community and heterosexual population.

DK Green is an advanced accredited psychotherapist and supervisor serving the GSRD (gender, sex and relationship diversity) communities that he co-inhabits. DK is an advanced trainer, associate lecturer, keynote speaker, webinar instructor and author for Pink Therapy; prolific presenter at Polyday, universities, NHS and many more; and founding member of http://polycounselling.co.uk. DK identifies as a queer, leather, polyamorous, spiritual, family transman.

Rima Hawkins is a COSRT and EMDR (UK) accredited, a Pink Therapy clinical associate and a UKCP registered sex and relationship psychotherapist, a trauma therapist and a supervisor. Her specialism is in cultural intersectionality, intimate and interpersonal violence and in pre-trial therapy (PTT). She's also an expert witness in court.

Dr Alex Iantaffi, PhD, MS, SEP, CST, LMFT (they/he/lui) is a family therapist, WPATH certified gender specialist, AASECT certified sex therapist, Somatic Experiencing® practitioner, clinical supervisor and award-winning author. They have researched, presented and published extensively on gender, disability, sexuality and relationships. More information available at www.alexiantaffi.com

Guillermo Llorca is an integrative psychosexual and relationship therapist. Originally from Spain, he developed his career in LGBT, mental health, HIV and sexual health sectors in London. He works relationally and creatively with different presentations including trauma, sexual abuse, shame, compulsive sexual behaviour, chemsex and issues specific to sexual diversity and orientation.

Ellis Morgan is a gender identity therapist in private practice in London. His writing includes collaborations with Strathclyde University and Scottish

Transgender Alliance 'Dangerous Education: The Occupational Hazards of Teaching Transgender' (2018) and 'Transforming Research Practice' (2016). He was previously a director within the LGBTQ+ mental health sector.

Joel Simpson is a UKCP registered psychotherapist, presenter, group facilitator, trainer, writer and celebrant. With a soulful intention to listen through the heart, Joel leads, speaks, teaches and writes with a reclaimed voice. As a celebrant, Joel crafts love-centred ceremonies for life's rites of passage, transitions and celebrations.

Foreword

Dr Meg-John Barker

As somebody who entered queer psychology, and began training as a therapist, in the early 2000s, the original Pink Therapy books had a huge impact on me. It's wonderful – two decades on – to see how the Pink Therapy community has gone from strength to strength with its events, international trainings, and impact, and to celebrate two new additions to the Pink Therapy book series – Silva and Dominic's collections *Erotically Queer* and *Relationally Queer*.

These books are a wonderful celebration of the work of the current wave of Pink Therapists, and an excellent reflection of what Pink Therapy has always done so well: moving with the rapidly changing times, and reflecting the full diversity of identities and experiences under the queer umbrella.

It pleases me, as someone who specialised as a sex and relationship therapist and now writes in these areas, that these collections have taken erotics and relationships as their focus. Together, the two books provide a much-needed up-to-date overview of the range of erotic practices and relationship styles for those working with queer clients. However, they do so much more than this.

A huge problem with both research and therapeutic practice around sex and relationships is the limited normative understanding these are embedded in which regards the erotic as penetrative sex leading to orgasm, and relationships as monogamous romantic couples. One of the deepest teachings of ace and aro communities is that the erotic is about far more than sex, and love is about far more than romance. We can find love and eroticism in the same – or different – places; we can find them with ourselves, with another person, with many others, and/or beyond the human realm (with land, or spirit, for example).

These books help all practitioners – whether working specifically with queer clients or not – to understand the rich diversity of eroticism and human relating which is possible, and present. It's vital that all therapists expand their understanding to encompass this range, rather than focusing on such limited aims as enabling erect penises and penetrable vaginas, or keeping romantic couples together in atomised units.

This book, *Relationally Queer*, does an excellent job of setting out the restrictive dominant cultural – and therapeutic – norms of relationships (Y Gávriel Ansara), and then exploring how we might work with those whose relationships challenge these norms. This encompasses LGBTQIA+ relationships in general

(Rima Hawkins), and Bi+ relationships specifically (Susannah Grant) which challenge both hetero- and homonormativity. It also encompasses consensually non-monogamous relationships of various kinds (DK Green), and couple relationships which trouble the monogamy/non-monogamy binary by being – to some degree – open (Niki D).

However, the norms that restrict our understandings and experiences of relationships go beyond hetero-, homo-, and mono-normativities. There is also what has been labelled amatonormativity: the assumption that romantic relationships are the most important kind of relationships which everyone should be pursuing, with other kinds of relationships regarded as somehow lesser. We see this in the assumption that 'relationship therapy' equates to 'marriage' or 'couple' therapy. Amatonormativity devalues the friendship, family-of-choice, and queer kinship relationships which are vital to so many LGTBQIA+ people and beyond. It's great to see such deep coverage here of relationships in and with community (Dominic Davies), and professional relationships between sex/relationship workers and their clients (Cyndi Darnell and Daniel Bąk).

I'm excited by the chapters in this book which touch on relationships beyond those between humans. Ellis Morgan presents a hugely helpful model for understanding trans people's relationships with *ourselves* – depending on whether we claim our gender or not, and whether we foreground our transness or not. Guillermo Llorca considers the impact of antiretroviral therapy on gay men's relationships with their bodies and themselves. Joel Simpson explores the relationship between queer African diasporan people and their homes, roots, and ancestors, in the context of violent colonialism and its ongoing legacy.

Finally, my sense is that we often become preoccupied with the question of *what* relationships people are engaged in (queer or straight, monogamous or non-monogamous, friendship or partnership, etc.) when what is far more vital is *how* people relate, connect, and love. Alex Iantaffi's chapter introduces the disability justice framework as an extremely helpful model for how we might all build more caring, sustainable, access-intimate, and trauma-sensitive relationships. Saquib Ahmad explores how faith and spirituality weave through LGBTQIA+ people's relationships with themselves and others in ways that can both contract and expand their possibilities.

Relationships are vital to consider in the context of the huge threats that face us as this book is being published. The interconnected crises of social injustice and climate crisis are all about traumatised and traumatising relating. They involve treating some people, beings, and land as if they were of lesser – or no – value: as possessions, as resources, as disposable. The only way that we can address these crises is through relationship: through reconnecting with ourselves, through developing less violent and traumatic modes of relating with others, through working collectively in solidarity, and through recognising our interconnectedness and interdependence with all other beings and with the land. This collection is an important contribution to the conversation about how we can begin to do (queer) relating differently.

Introduction

Silva Neves and Dominic Davies

It is undeniable that connections and relationships are central to our well-being. Relationships of all kinds are good for us: friendships, peers, intimate relationships and supportive colleagues. It could be argued that connections and relationships are even more essential for us Queer people because we live in a heteronormative, mononormative, sex-negative and cisgenderist world that can often obstruct us in making such connections and finding each other. Faced with ongoing discrimination, stigmatisation, marginalisation and exclusion, Queer people mustn't live in isolation. We need to build up trusted social networks, which have been called "tribe" or "team" or "logical family" (Maupin, 2017), rather than biological family, which may comprise supportive family members, friends, colleagues, allies, casual lovers and long-term intimate partners.

Our biggest wounds happen in relationships when someone who is supposed to love and care for us hurts us, betrays us or abuses us. It could be our parents, close friends, family members or lovers. In addition to these more intimate relationships, the Queer community has its fair share of wounds from the outside world. Homophobia, biphobia, transphobia and sexophobia are relational traumas that can deeply wound us, especially when it comes from people who should be offering us a safe space. No child should be afraid of their parents if they do not conform to cisgender monogamous heterosexuality. No child should be bullied in their school for being "different". Nobody should be discriminated against when accessing healthcare. Nobody should worry about holding their same-sex partner's hand in the streets. But here we are, a world full of hate crimes against Queer people. Having a "tribe" is where we get to help each other and learn the skills to navigate this imperfect world.

Having a "tribe", being in good intimate relationships, and having a supportive social network are fundamental human rights. Still, it is hard to achieve, especially if we have never learned to love ourselves, never understood our worth, and instead have internalised negative core beliefs about ourselves, believing that we don't deserve what is readily available for cisgender, monogamous, heterosexual people: consistent respect, visibility, a safe environment, and legal and institutional protections to live our lives.

DOI: 10.4324/9781003260561-1

This book is about Queer intimate relationships, but you will see that it is also about genuine human connections, great compassion and deep love for our Queer communities. Our authors aim to help therapists work with our diverse Queer relationships by offering new ideas and contemporary methods, adapting theory to be more GSRD-friendly, cutting-edge thinking and challenging the status quo of *couple therapy* which is rooted in heteronormative and mononormative thinking. Can we encourage you all to use the term *relationship therapy*?

We know that the most crucial part of therapy is the therapeutic relationship. We have a special relationship with our clients, a meaningful connection in which we are responsible for creating a safe place. We must never forget it because, as stated earlier, we can deeply wound someone in the therapeutic relationship if we don't maintain a safe space. This requires us to learn, continually practise cultural humility (Stubbe, 2020) and engage with GSRD-sensitive supervision and our therapy.

We don't believe in the binary of good and bad therapists. We think most therapists are well-intentioned and in this profession for the right reason. Unfortunately, many therapists are let down by an absence of experiential training to raise their self-awareness, learning core GSRD theories, and deconstructing cis-het-mono normative frameworks which may not meet the specific needs of our Queer clients. Because of misinformation and poor training, therapists can accidentally end up harming clients within the therapeutic space. This book is our commitment to ending this.

As therapists, and especially when working with the Queer communities, we frequently hear awful stories of homophobia, biphobia, transphobia and slut-shaming; the trauma of growing up Queer in a straight world; the survivors of conversion practices; the ongoing minority stress; and all the Shadows of our clients. Of course, our job is to be with our clients in the dark moments. But we must not forget that surviving this world is not all about identifying Queer people. We must remember that we, too, deserve the best that life can offer. We can successfully integrate all the parts of ourselves to experience joy. Not only the pleasure of living in our "tribe" as a minority population but full-on Queer Joy.

Professor Esben Esther Pirelli Benestad discusses the terms "Transgifted", "Trans Joy" and "Trans Euphoria" in their excellent TED Talk as a way to think of ourselves from a strengths position. We can extend this sentiment to the entire Queer community.

Queer people have a long history of the "logical family", or "chosen family", in which we found much strength. When male homosexuality was illegal in Britain, we invented our secret language, Polari.[1]

Queer Joy is unapologetically embracing who we are, what we identify with, what we stand for and what brings meaning to our lives. It is not feeling like a minority because we compare ourselves to the "majority". For example, as gay men, we may dress more flamboyantly as an expression of our individuality and a challenge to toxic masculine hegemony. Here's an insightful contribution from a lesbian colleague, Maria Kindstedt:

I would say the number one thing lesbian is for me is freedom. And I don't mean personally, for me, being free to live as I do, but freedom in being a human being.

There are SO many expectations on cishet women and how to behave in relationships with men. There are so many unspoken codes of conduct and cultural expectations in EVERYTHING, personality, behaviour, sexual preferences, looks, courting etc. You are freer to be a person in a lesbian relationship. You are free to explore gender roles, gender, sexuality, courtship, love, friendships, and everything in relation-life is freer and safer as a lesbian.

With the lesbian desire of women comes respect for the feminine and feminine power. And yes, some lesbians enact toxic masculinity, etc. But I don't think there is anyone who truly loves women and the feminine in the way lesbians do.

This hidden resistance to the toxic patriarchal culture is almost like a place where the female and the feminine get centre stage and the entire stage for love and worship. It is quite beautiful and very empowering.

Queer Joy is not about feeling that we're "tolerated" in society. Being tolerated implies that the cis-het society "accommodates" us. We are not seeking approval or to be tolerated and deemed acceptable by the majority.

Queer Joy is about pridefully stepping into our power and asserting: *We Are Here*. No justification, explanation or apology is needed.

Queer people are gifted. There are many lessons or gifts we can offer heterosexual, monogamous, cisgender people:

- Asexual people teach us that desire has many forms and faces. All relationships can be equally significant rather than a hierarchy where a sexual relationship is deemed more important. Being together without sex can be just as pleasurable. They gift us the thinking that relationships are more unencumbered and more genuine when not motivated by covert or repressed desires.
- Lesbians empower women of all sexualities to challenge patriarchy by not caring about the male gaze, demonstrating how to be their own people without male approval. They also tend to have way more orgasms than women having sex with men.
- The Kink community has gifted us with the opportunity to widen our sexual repertoire and explore the recesses of our fantasy worlds, along with the art of clear conversation about our wants and needs and negotiating consent, which is now being followed up by the non-kink communities.
- Queer parents help their heterosexual counterparts expand their horizons with different ways of parenting outside of patriarchy, where childcare roles are more equally divided, and there is a much more thorough consideration of what it takes to have a child (because there are no unwanted pregnancies amongst Queer people).

- Our Consensual Non-Monogamists gift the world with the idea of compersion, challenging the reductive thinking of possessive jealousy.
- It's rare to find a gay male or lesbian couple objecting to their partner's use of pornography (apart from perhaps different preferences in porn). It teaches us not to "yuck another person's yum".
- Our pansexual friends show us how love and desire go beyond the genitals of their lovers, it's the whole person who matters, not what's between their legs. This can teach us to love more holistically.

We believe GSRD-informed Relationship Therapy can help many of our clients experience Queer Joy as part of their therapeutic journey because, as the worst wounds happen in relationships, the best healing also happens. Helping clients love themselves and have joyful, honest, open, intimate relationships is a key component of well-being.

Queer Joy is not an excuse to brush the hurt, wounds and trauma under the carpet and pretend to be happy. It's not about shouting, "*I'm out, I'm proud, all is fine*". We're not advocating for toxic positivity and denying the very real struggles many of us face daily. It is about acknowledging the pain, looking after ourselves, and aspiring to survive *and* thrive. Meyer (2015) speaks about resilience emerging from minority stress, and Dunlop (2022) offers ways to help each other with coping flexibly.

As GSRD practitioners, we are subject to vicarious trauma, both from hearing our clients' stories and what is happening in the world to our people. Connecting to our "tribe" is where we can nurture each other and is one strategy for maintaining good mental health.

Note

1 Polari was a language widely used by British gay men prior to the decriminalisation of male homosexuality in 1967 (www.babbel.com/en/magazine/what-is-polari). One can even find the King James Bible translated into Polari (www.polaribible.org/).

References

Dunlop, B. J. (2022). *The Queer Mental Health Handbook*. London: Jessica Kingsley Publisher.

Esben Esther Pirelli Benestad TED Talk. Retrieved from www.youtube.com/watch?v=H6blufLgo_U

Maupin, A. (2017). *Logical Family: A Memoir*. Transworld Publishers. London.

Meyer, I. H. (2015). Resilience in the study of minority stress and health of sexual and gender minorities. *Psychology of Sexual Orientation and Gender Diversity*, 2(3), 209–213.

Stubbe, D. (2020). Practicing cultural competence and cultural humility in the care of diverse patients. *Focus*, 18(1), 49–51. https://doi.org/10.1176/appi.focus.20190041

Chapter 1

Getting real about monogamism

Disrupting mononormative bias in sex therapy and relationship counselling

Dr Y Gávriel Ansara

Monogamism (Anderson, 2010; cf. Twist et al., 2018) is the belief that monogamous people and relationships are superior, more mature, or more "natural", while polyamorous and multi-partnered relationships are inferior, inherently unstable, immature, less "committed", or "unnatural". Mononormativity (Pieper & Bauer, 2005) refers to the societal standard of monogamy that frames relationships in terms of a monogamy/"infidelity" binary. *Couple-centric bias* is the widespread mononormative bias that all people have or should desire a "couple" relationship.

This chapter explores ways to identify and disrupt mononormative bias in sex therapy and relationship counselling with polyamorous and multi-partnered people. I use the term "polyamorous and multi-partnered" people to acknowledge that people with polyamorous lived experiences are not necessarily partnered and that people with multiple partners may or may not self-identify as polyamorous. Additional forms of erotic and intimate connection are beyond the scope of this chapter. My social position in writing this chapter is as a polyamorous person and sex and relationship therapist with over a decade of experience in providing clinical guidance and therapeutic support alongside polyamorous people, kinship systems, and communities.

Monogamist forms of epistemic injustice

Fricker (2007) delineated two forms of epistemic injustice: testimonial injustice and hermeneutical injustice. According to Fricker, *testimonial injustice* occurs when people's accounts of their lived experiences are treated as less credible due to their marginalised status (e.g., a polyamorous parent is viewed as having a less credible account of parenting than a monogamous parent, partially or entirely due to societal stigma against polyamorous people). *Hermeneutical injustice* describes challenges in understanding people's lived experiences, when such descriptions have been historically excluded from the collective explanatory resources people use to make sense of their lived experiences (e.g., when polyamorous people have difficulty explaining their lived experiences due to not having prior exposure to language about polyamorous dynamics and emotional responses).

Hermeneutical injustice against polyamorous and multi-partnered people pervades the professions of sex therapy, relationship counselling, and family therapy.

DOI: 10.4324/9781003260561-2

Virtually all assessments used in relationship and family therapy have been designed for, and tested only on, married woman/man dyads (Kisler & Lock, 2019). Most sex and relationship therapy studies are either influenced by unscientific biases about polyamorous relationships or exclude polyamorous people entirely (Girard & Brownlee, 2015). The leading relationship counselling approaches promote couple-centric frameworks that reinforce monogamism and exclude key concepts for respectful and effective relationship therapy with polyamorous and multi-partnered people and polycules (see definition on p.9). Even polyamorous and multi-partnered therapists have not been adequately prepared for clinical assessment and therapeutic work involving polyamorous and multi-partnered relationship systems.

Critical reflection on mononormative biases

Due to the aforementioned forms of hermeneutical injustice, many therapists have difficulty even identifying their own deeply entrenched mononormative biases. Kean (2018) addressed this gap by identifying 11 mononormative biases:

- The passionate/romantic ideal of "one true love".
- The steady/companionate ideal of a "soul mate".
- The idea that the measure of commitment is sexual "fidelity".
- The idea that the measure of commitment is emotional "fidelity".
- The fact that "fidelity" and "faithfulness" are understood as synonyms of "monogamy".
- The belief that having one sexual-romantic partner at a time is mature/natural/best.
- The idea that there is a clear, coherent, and sustainable distinction between the categories of "friend" and "lover".
- The belief that sex is healthy only in the company of romance and commitment.
- The way romance and commitment are understood as leading to or synonymous with monogamy.
- The belief that sex means you are serious about someone.
- The contradictory belief that sex with more than one person shows you are not serious about those people.

Kean's longer version of this list delineates 50 mononormative biases (Kean, 2015, pp. 700–702). This list of 50 mononormative biases can be a valuable audit tool for practitioners wishing to conduct a mononormative bias inventory of their own clinical practice. Practitioners can also use these lists to guide solo and relationship therapy participants through critical self-reflection and serve as clinically beneficial disruptions to unexamined mononormative biases. However, practitioners must first examine and address our own mononormative biases before achieving the congruence and self-awareness necessary for this nuanced clinical work.

Mononormative vocabularies of emotion

The harmful impact of therapists' mononormative biases is well-established (e.g., Cassidy & Wong, 2018; Grunt-Mejer & Łyś, 2019; Henrich & Trawinski, 2016; Jordan, 2018; Kisler & Lock, 2019; van Tol, 2017). Vocabularies of emotion can be mechanisms for enacting mononormative social control (Harré & Parrott, 1996). Ritchie and Barker (2006) asserted that the construction of jealousy as a "natural" response to "infidelity" and a "negative" emotion perpetuates mononormative bias. Mononormative characterisations of jealousy neglect the therapeutic reasoning needed to distinguish between a monogamous person who is dissatisfied with their existing relationship *partner* and an ostensibly monogamous but actually polyamorous person who may be dissatisfied with their monogamous relationship *configuration*. Despite the central focus on "infidelity", "cheating", and "affairs" in relationship counselling, few of the major schools of relationship therapy have adequately acknowledged or addressed this distinction or taught the essential nature of investigating whether the monogamous aspect of the relationship agreement itself was established with mutual informed consent and discussion of multiple options, instead of being based on the coercive control dynamic of non-consensual or compulsory monogamy (see Heckert, 2010; Robinson, 2013).

Although extensive research has documented securely attached and emotionally mature polyamorous kinships, many relationship therapists have been taught that polyamorous relationships result from poor impulse control, insecure attachment, or emotional immaturity. Due to this stereotype, therapists routinely presume that an ostensibly monogamous person who engages in romantic or erotic intimacy outside of their monogamous relationship has made "a mistake", or "strayed", or that they or their monogamous relationship must be deficient. In a polycule-centred framework, therapists responding to so-called "infidelity" investigate whether monogamy was explicitly agreed upon or assumed and whether a new agreement needs to be negotiated to incorporate emerging needs and desires.

Therapists' failure to recognise polyamorous and multi-partnered people and relationship configurations is a clinical problem that endangers our ability to make accurate clinical judgements or achieve optimal clinical outcomes (Jordan, 2018). To address hermeneutical injustice, therapists must consider the implicit ideology of our language about emotions and the extent to which we integrate polyamorous and multi-partnered vocabularies and concepts. Although some cultures and societies already have traditional terms and concepts to describe multi-partnered relationship systems, Ritchie and Barker (2006) documented how English-speaking polyamorous communities in a mononormative society needed to develop new language to describe their identities, define their relationships, and express their emotions. They noted that vocabularies of emotion ascribe value and meaning to emotions and are therefore inherently ideological. Before practitioners can support people with expressing and processing their experiences, we need to share a more inclusive language of emotions (see Barker, 2005).

Mononormative vocabularies of emotion entrench couple-centric bias and limit clinical conceptualisations of romantic and erotic connections outside of dyads ("couples") to mononormative concepts such as "infidelity" and "adultery". Research suggests having romantic and/or sexual interactions with more than one person is much more common than therapists may presume (e.g., Haupert et al., 2017). Multiple studies have documented that at least 20% (and, in some studies, up to 70%) of ostensibly monogamous, married people have engaged in romantic and/or erotic interactions with additional partners, a finding that highlights the permeability and incongruity of the mono/polyam binary (see Kipnis, 1998, particularly footnote 4, p. 293).

Ritchie and Barker's (2006) participants described a polyamorous emotion called *compersion* as "an exact antonym of jealousy" (George, 1997, cited in Ritchie & Barker, 2006, p. 595), "taking joy in one's partner's other partners" (Cathy, 2000, cited in ibid.), or "the feeling of taking joy in the joy that others you love share among themselves, especially taking joy in the knowledge that your beloveds are expressing their love for one another" (moderators of the LiveJournal Compersion community in 2003, as cited in ibid.). Other participants disliked compersion because "it somehow brings to mind the two words . . . compelled and coercion", preferring the term *frubbly* due to being "all in favour of a 'snuggly' word" (Jane, 2000, cited in ibid.). This contrast highlights the diversity of emotional vocabularies among English-speaking multi-partnered relationships.

Subsequent studies support Ritchie and Barker's (2006) finding that monogamous people need different vocabularies of emotion than polyamorous people. In a survey, Ritchie and Barker asked 529 monogamous people and 159 polyamorous and multi-partnered people to share their reactions to imagining their romantic partner with another partner. Monogamous partners reported greater emotional distress than polyamorous and multi-partnered people. Polyamorous and multi-partnered people reported thinking about their partner's other partners more frequently, and they were more likely to report positive emotional responses to imagining their romantic partner with another partner – including reactions consistent with compersion (see Mogilski et al., 2019 for complete findings, but see Hyde, 2005, for a feminist critique of this kind of "gender differences" approach and how this gender ideology can affect both research findings and researchers' interpretations of their findings). Mogilski et al.'s (2019) findings highlight the dangers of assuming the universality of monogamous emotional and communication norms and substantiate the need for practitioners to apply a polycule-centred vocabulary of emotions in therapeutic contexts.

Unfortunately, some of the most popular introductory texts on polyamorous and multi-partnered relationships contain mononormative biases (see Ansara, 2020 for a list of useful educational resources). Therapists must reflect on how the vocabularies of emotion we invoke in therapeutic contexts can enact monogamist erasure of some people's emotional experiences (Cassidy & Wong, 2018). Well-intentioned empathy cannot replace the expertise and skill that come from lived experience; for monogamous therapists, cultural humility (Tervalon & Murray-García, 1998) can establish safer therapeutic environments than unsustainable claims of cultural competence. Polyamorous and multi-partnered people need therapists to be comfortable and familiar with using polyamorous vocabularies of emotion in clinical practice (Ritchie & Barker, 2006). This need for fluency in polycule-centred language may be one of the reasons why many polyamorous and multi-partnered people have reported having better experiences with therapists who are polyamorous and/or multi-partnered than with therapists who are monogamous. Monogamous therapists can be most successful when they acknowledge and criti-cally reflect on how mononormative privilege can limit their understanding. It is difficult to conceal one's relative unfamiliarity and discomfort with polyamorous vocabularies of emotion. To address this limitation, monogamous practitioners can educate themselves through exposure to a range of polyamorous communities and lived experience narratives outside of sessions and can express cultural humility both within and beyond sessions by acknowledging that polyamorous and multi-partnered people are the best authorities to consult about our own lives.

Using polyamorous vocabularies of emotion and experience can promote greater visibility and understanding. The term *polycule* describes all people within a multi-partnered kinship system as a kind of polyamorous "molecule" (Creation, 2019; Fern, 2020; Sheff & Wolf, 2015). Polycules can also include monogamous partners of a polyamorous partner in the system. Terms such as *pod, bubble,* and *House* are sometimes preferred to the term *family,* which some multi-partnered people consider exclusionary. The term family also has discriminatory connota-tions that stem from its history of being weaponised in political campaigns that have targeted people outside of heteronormative nuclear families. Where the term "family" is used, qualifiers can be added (e.g., *found* family, *chosen* family, family *of origin,* or *bio* family) to avoid the default privileging of some familial bonds over others (see also Kaldera, 2005; Kean, 2018). Polyamorous kinship systems, particularly polyamorous parents, have yet to be adequately addressed within the field of family therapy or even recognised as legitimate forms of families, despite some promising developments by some polyamorous family and parenting researchers (e.g., Pallotta-Chiarolli et al., 2020). For example, in response to my presentation on working with polyamorous families at a national family therapy peak body, one family therapist said that although they had enjoyed my presenta-tion, it was "not about families" and "not relevant to family therapy". This kind of monogamist bias is an example of how the term "family" is often defined by family therapists in ways that exclude and discriminate against polyamorous and multi-partnered people and our kinship systems.

Attachments that matter

Some people practise *hierarchical polyamory,* in which partners are ranked in terms of their relative closeness and primacy (e.g., "primary partner", "sec-ondary partner"). In contrast, some polyamorous people practise *egalitarian polyamory,* often termed *non-hierarchical polyamory.* Some people consider hierarchical approaches inherently oppressive, stifling, or dehumanising due to the hierarchical privilege granted to some partners. Some of the most intractable relationship conflicts can occur between polyamorous partners who disagree regarding whether their relationships should have a hierarchical or egalitarian structure. It is essential to be aware that structure alone does not determine the relative quality or oppressiveness of a particular relationship sub-system within a polycule; what matters more is the extent to which the needs of all polycule members are prioritised and adequately addressed. Fern (2020) described the ideal polyamorous relational state of *polysecurity* as one in which all polycule members can experience the multi-partnered relationship system as a safe haven and a secure attachment base.

The terms *solo polyamory* and *single polyamory* are each used in a variety of contrasting context-dependent ways, sometimes treated as distinct and sometimes used interchangeably. Depending on context, these terms may refer to polyamorous people who do not wish to engage in any erotic or romantic commitments; people who wish to have erotic and/or romantic connections but avoid "couple" status, cohabitation, and/or hierarchical relationships (e.g., *primary*, *secondary*, and other categories for rank-ordering one's partners); people who view themselves as their own primary partner; and people who prioritise emotional intimacy rather than romantic and/or erotic relational components when determining the value and primacy of their relationships (see Fern, 2020, pp. 114–115 for discussion of some common misconceptions regarding solo polyamory).

The related concept of *relationship anarchy* (Nordgren, 2006) describes an adaptation of political anarchist principles applied to interpersonal relationships. Although this term is often misused to describe all non-hierarchical multi-partnered relationships, Fern (2020) explained that

> relationship anarchists seek to dismantle the social hierarchies dictating how sexual and romantic relationships are prioritized over all other forms of love, and so people who identify as relationship anarchists make less distinction between the importance or value of their lovers over their friends or other people in their life, and they do not only reserve intimacy or romance for the people they have sex with.
>
> (p. 115)

Popular media representations of polyamory typically exclude people on the aromantic (aro) and asexual (ace) spectra, some of whom engage in romance and/ or erotic activities under some conditions. Definitions of polyamory that centre on romantic and erotic intimacy can devalue or exclude people on the aro and/or ace spectrum who seek secure interpersonal attachments primarily through emotional rather than romantic or erotic forms of intimacy. Relationship anarchy has the potential to subvert the social hierarchies that devalue aro and ace spectrum people's interpersonal attachments. To achieve inclusive practice with aro and ace spectrum people, practitioners must recognise and affirm that romantic and erotic forms of intimacy are not universal indicators of relationship quality.

Kean (2018, 2015) critiqued attempts to disentangle sex and love in a consistent manner across a diversity of relationship configurations and interrogated the politics of delineating interpersonal categories and relationship valuations. Kean reminded readers that

> it is crucial to recognise that while these inconsistencies within mononormativity become apparent in the context of the non-monogamous sex/love skirmishes described in this article, the skirmishes do not cause the inconsistencies. Practitioners of different kinds of non-monogamy jostling for position in relation to mainstream practices of sex, love, and friendship simply elucidate the fact that the relational logics that sustain those practices only ever partially cohere.
>
> (Kean, 2018, p. 13)

Challenging everyday monogamism means recognising the social relations of power at play in these culturally mononormative naming and meaning-making processes and avoiding relational logics that grant therapists the authority to determine each person's relative value and meaning in the relational system. Consider how therapists might misconstrue (which involve infrequent contact) or fail to grasp the significance of a *queerplatonic relationship (QPR)*, an intimate and intense relationship with diverse and sometimes conflicting definitions that cannot be adequately defined within a "friend versus lover" binary (Coyote, 2019). Furthermore, Kean (2018) indicated that the goal of achieving coherent relational logic and distinctions (e.g., friend versus lover) might itself be inherently problematic and unattainable.

Polyamory means different things to different people (Klesse, 2011; Klesse, 2014b). Where polyamory is, for some people, a behaviour (e.g., Barker, 2005), for others, it is a lifestyle and identity (e.g., Henrich & Trawinski, 2016) or a relational orientation (e.g., Jordan, 2018). Some people define polyamory as a relationship philosophy (Klesse, 2013), a political stance, or a way of approaching the relational dimension of life (e.g., Anapol, 2010; Nordgren, 2006). By focussing on the diversity of polyamorous and multi-partnered people's lived experiences and kinship bonds instead of on abstract theoretical constructs, practitioners can prioritise the feelings and needs of actual polyamorous and multi-partnered people, relationships, and communities.

Everyday mononormative concepts

Therapists trained in mononormative relationship therapy approaches are often unaware that describing their scope of practice as "couples counselling" unintentionally communicates an unwillingness to work with people in multi-partnered relational systems. Conceptualising relationship therapy work solely in terms of "couples" can also impair therapists' diagnostic reasoning. Therapists primed by couple-centric concepts may omit pivotal questions and considerations when exploring people's relationship and attachment histories. By limiting the scope of relationship therapy to "couples", therapists may also overlook the often crucial need to include *metamours* (people who share one or more partner[s] in common without being designated romantic or erotic partners to each other) in psychosocial history taking, in relationship assessments, and in the core tasks of relationship therapy.

Where metamours are included, therapists often relegate them to the marginalised or demonised status of "the other woman/man/person". Metamours play pivotal roles in many polyamorous and multi-partnered people's lives, with some metamour relationships having equal importance to romantic and erotic partnerships. Some metamour relationships can shift into romantic and/or erotic partnerships while people continue their relationships with their shared partners. Some metamour relationships develop and deepen following relationship dissolution with a previously shared romantic and/or erotic partner. Given the diverse permutations within polycules, it is vital for therapists to consider metamours as integral to the relational system and to value metamours' insights regarding the relationships within their polycule.

In relationship and family therapy, genograms are widely used visual tools through which therapists use codes and symbols to obtain and communicate detailed information about the composition, dynamics, and patterns in kinship systems. In addition, genograms can illustrate affective, behavioural, and cognitive components. Genograms have also been used as a therapeutic assessment method and as a form of "intervention" (McGoldrick et al., 2008). Genograms created by polyamorous and multi-partnered people typically prioritise information that is excluded from the mononormative, couple-centric genograms with which most therapists are familiar.

Mononormative genograms represent people with symbols based on their gender, whereas polyam-generated genograms often limit gender references to pronoun(s) use or omit gender entirely. Conversely, polyam-generated genograms often contain information missing from mononormative genograms. Polycule-centred genograms typically identify relationship dynamics such as *nesting partners* (a common polyamorous term for cohabiting partners in an egalitarian polyamorous kinship system), metamours, former lovers, asexual romances, queerplatonic relationships, long-distance relationships, people with shared parenting/child caregiving roles, people who share finances or projects, and people who are considering becoming lovers (e.g., Wolf, 2013, 2015, 2016). Some hierarchical polycules construct genograms that delineate primary and secondary partners, relationships between monogamous and polyamorous partners, relationship anarchists, and people who practise solo polyamory. Some polyam genograms identify monogamous people within the polycule, whereas a mononormative genogram would simply assume monogamous status. Several websites allow people to create their own polycule genograms (e.g., https://polycul.es/create). Within polyamorous social networks, it is common for new and prospective partners to share polycule genograms or similar diagrams to facilitate clear communication about their existing relationship systems and kinship bonds.

Whereas monogamist notions of relational systems presume that all sub-systems take the form of dyads, some polycules consist of triadic, quadratic, or other structures without any dyads. This includes *triads* (three people who are all relationship partners to each other), *quads* (four people in a relationship with each other), and *Vs* also known as *pivots*, *anchors*, or *hinges* (two partners with a shared partner in common who are each other's metamours).

Many well-intentioned therapists refer to polyamorous people as living "alterna-tive lifestyles" or as "non-traditional". Yet polyamorous people come from all walks of life and may lead conventional or conservative lifestyles. From a cross-cultural and historical perspective, the contemporary couple relationship is the "alternative lifestyle". The ethnocentric bias in referring to relationships with more than two people as "non-traditional" is evident when one considers cultures and societies where formal recognition of multiple partners has been and continues to be "tradi-tional" (e.g., Benedict, 2017; Du, 2016; Legros, 2014; Zeitzen, 2020). Cross-cultural analyses reveal that monogamy is not merely a neutral and universally normative social construct but a culturally specific, settler-colonial construct embedded with the racialisation, ethnocentrism, and ableism of its historical roots. When a therapist uses the phrase "alternative lifestyle", their assumption that all people in polyamorous and multi-partnered relationship systems are living a particular "lifestyle" and that they are countercultural in some way reinforces ethnocentric and racist ideology.

Researchers have documented age, income, gender, sexuality, culture, and racialised demographic category diversity among polyamorous people and rela-tionships (Moors et al., 2014; Rubin et al., 2014). Some people in polyamorous kinship systems are part of particular religious, cultural, and subcultural com-munities, whereas others are part of the dominant cultural group in their region. Multi-partnered people come from across the political and socioeconomic spec-trum. Multi-partnered people can experience unique socioeconomic inequalities due to the impact of intersecting racialised and class-based oppression on their options for accessing and navigating intimacy and care, household formation, and spaces and institutions (Klesse, 2014a). Some polyamorous and multi-partnered people have experienced intersecting racism, classism, and other forms of sys-temic oppression within polyamorous communities (Sheff & Hammers, 2011; see Manduley, 2015). Some multi-partnered people are parents; some are therapists. No single lifestyle or way of life is common to people with polyamorous and/or multi-partnered lived experience, so-called "alternative" or otherwise.

Despite recent increases in the number of countries that recognise dyadic same-gender: dyadic same-gender marriages for people with binary woman or man administrative gender designations – and, in some jurisdictions such as Australia, recognition for non-binary people's marriages – there is only limited and heavily gendered formal recognition for multi-partnered relationships worldwide. A vari-ety of countries recognise the right of men within particular religious and cultural communities to have multiple spouses as long as they marry women. According to anthropological records, about 85% of human societies have permitted men to marry multiple women (Henrich et al., 2012). Fewer jurisdictions currently permit women and non-binary people to have multiple spouses of any gender. In the matrilineal Naxi or Na (often called Moso or Mósuō) society in southwestern China, it is traditional practice for women to have multiple *tisese* or "walking back and forth" relationships with *acia*, partners who live in separate dwellings (Du, 2016; Hua, 2001; Shih, 2000). There is no traditional term for "husband" or "father" in Na society (Hua, 2001; Shih, 2000). Historically, these multi-partnered relationships did not involve contractual agreements, binding obligations, or exclusivity, although some of these aspects of tisese relationships have shifted in recent decades in some Na communities that have had more contact with other cultures (Shih, 2000).

In 2012, in Rio de Janeiro, Brazil, Public Notary Claudia do Nascimento Domingues provided official state recognition for the civil union between a triad of two women and a man, despite vocal criticism by some religious organisations (BBC News, 2012). In the United States, the suburban city of Somerville in Massachusetts has formally recognised simultaneously registered partnerships with multiple partners since June 2020 (Fox, 2020). Somerville is currently one of the only places in the world that offers something approaching – but not fully equal to – equitable relationship recognition for people of all genders in multi-partnered kinship systems.

Since at least the 1990s, the term "marriage equality" has become synonymous with the movement for legal recognition of civil marriages between two monogamous partners with the same gender marker on their government-issued identity documents (e.g., Marriage Equality USA, n.d.). Therapists familiar with struggles for dyadic same-gender marriage recognition sometimes use the phrase "marriage equality" when discussing people's legislative rights and options for relationship recognition. Unfortunately, this misleading phrase functions to erase the ongoing lack of equitable relationship rights for people in polyamorous relationships and multi-partnered kinship systems.

In many jurisdictions, there is still profound marriage inequality and blatant, state-sanctioned discrimination against people in multi-partnered kinship systems. Many people in multi-partnered relationships face the agonising choice regarding whether to gain legal protections and marriage recognition with one partner while risking the devaluing of all other partners or to forgo marriage benefits with any one partner to prevent discrimination against their other relationships. Polyamorous and multi-partnered people also experience immigration discrimination. Many countries have partnership visa eligibility requirements that deny access to people in polyamorous and multi-partnered relationships. In some countries, people with partner visas can face deportation, criminal fraud charges, and state-sanctioned abuse if they are discovered to be polyamorous or multi-partnered (Jenkins & Rickert, 2020; Klesse, 2016). In many countries, polyamorous people can lose or be denied custody of their children or face criminal charges and state-sanctioned abuse solely due to being polyamorous or multi-partnered (Jenkins &

Rickert, 2020; Klesse, 2019; Pallotta-Chiarolli et al., 2020). Therapists who recognise these legitimate concerns can avoid unwitting complicity with state-sanctioned abuse of polyamorous and multi-partnered people. In such cases, it is important to recognise the anti-oppressive practice principle that advocacy is a professional duty when working with people with lived experience of oppression and marginalisation (Brown, 2019).

The term "consensual non-monogamies" (CNM) is often used where a similar qualifier is not used to describe monogamy as "consensual". This linguistic disparity can obscure ubiquitous forms of non-consensual monogamy, such as compulsory and coerced monogamy (e.g., Wilkinson, 2012). This selective use of the qualifier "consensual" also places polyamorous and multi-partnered relationships under inherent moral suspicion for consent violations, despite the well-established ethical norms for consent, negotiation, and boundaries in polyamorous communities. This inequitable framing also obscures polyamorous community norms centred around ethical principles such as honesty, communication, consent, respectful negotiation, and integrity (Barker & Langdridge, 2010). A polycule-centred approach can recognise polyamorous relationships and kinship systems as distinct phenomena without disproportionate use of a moral qualifier (e.g., "consensual") or comparisons to a monogamous reference point (e.g., "non-monogamy").

As clarified by various authors (e.g., Cohen, 2016; Matsick et al., 2014; Conley, in Naftulin, 2019), open monogamy is distinct from polyamory. The term "open monogamy" typically refers to couple-centric, dyadic relationships in which two partners formally agree to engage in romantic and/or erotic connections with other people while maintaining couple privilege and primacy. This is distinct from polyamory, which does not automatically presume that any two people in a multi-partnered relationship agree or desire to privilege their dyadic bond as superior to, or more important than, their other partner relationships. Fern (2020) observed that polyamorous representations in English language formats up to the early 2000s highlighted hierarchical polyamorous relationships and described multi-partner relationships in terms of primary and secondary partners. This focus on hierarchical polyamorous relationships and the use of couple-centric terminology to describe multiple partners (e.g., "extra-pair relationships" in Mogilski et al., 2019) persists in contemporary research. Hierarchical bias also pervades commonly recommended introductory educational resources on polyamorous and multi-partner relationships. In the foreword to Fern (2020), author Eve Rickert acknowledges that Rickert's co-authored critique of hierarchical polyamorous relationships

> fell short. It placed the onus of building security almost entirely on the individual who felt insecure. Despite the many people who were helped by the book, this inappropriate focus caused harm, and over time, I grew to understand there was something missing in our framework – I just didn't have the words for what.
>
> (Rickert, in Fern, 2020, p. x, para. 3)

This hermeneutical injustice is part of why many therapists struggle to distinguish between polyamorous and open relationships. Polycule-centred practice interrogates the power and privilege dynamics that can occur when a monogamous dyad invites additional partners into a pre-existing, couple-centric relationship while preserving the original couple-privileged hierarchy and retaining agreements that were not equitably co-authored by everyone in the polycule.

Polyamorous relationships are not necessarily "open"; the term *polyfidelitous* is often used to designate a closed polyamorous relationship system or polycule. An "open monogamy stance" differs from a polycule-centred practice, which values all relationships within a polycule. To avoid harming our participants, therapists need to transcend dyadic thinking that presumes all relationships have a dyad at their base.

One pervasive monogamist assumption is that a monogamous dyad who wish to shift into a multi-partnered relational system can do so while maintaining the exact same dynamic, core agreements, and boundaries of their pre-existing monogamous relationship. This approach can endanger the wellbeing of all people in the relational system. In Fern (2020), Eve Rickert noted that the hierarchical frameworks in media representations such as *Polyamorous: Married and Dating*

> did a dismal job of honouring the attachment needs of partners who were considered "secondary": those outside a primary, usually presumed to be nesting, couple, whose bond was presumed to be more valid or worthy of protection than the others "opened up" to.
>
> (Rickert, in Fern, 2020, p. ix)

The original relationship can only meet the needs of additional, newer polycule members by giving those new members an opportunity to communicate, negotiate, and change the previously established dynamic. Denying new polycule members this right violates the ethical norms of polyamorous communities (e.g., Barker & Langdridge, 2010). The default hierarchical structure of open, couple-centred relationships requires specific attention to ensure that the attachment-related needs of newer partners are adequately addressed (Fern, 2020).

Autonomy vs. permission norms

Polyamorous community norms about romantic and erotic intimacy and relationship status vary widely. Although relational categories are inherently fraught, permeable, and contested (Heckert, 2010; Kean, 2018; Klesse, 2006; Robinson, 2013), establishing clear and consensual boundaries is vital to relational safety and autonomy. In my therapeutic practice, I have identified two contrasting ethical boundary norms within polyamorous and multi-partnered communities and relationships: the *autonomy norm*, which holds that all people have a default right to unconstrained autonomy in their erotic and romantic activities, and the *permission norm*, which holds that partners have a default right to expect erotic and

romantic exclusivity unless given specific approval. In the autonomy norm, partners are free to engage in romantic and erotic intimacy and to contract relationships in any manner they choose unless they have given explicit consent to limit
this behaviour or consult with partners before making decisions. Conversely, in
the permission norm, partners set limits on their partners' romantic or erotic intimacy with other people. This means one partner expects another partner not to
engage in romantic or erotic behaviour outside their relationship unless they have
given explicit permission.

Mononormative counselling approaches typically presume the moral superior-
ity of the permission norm. This presumption can undermine a crucial task of
relationship therapists, which is to assist people in identifying and communicating about the norms underlying relational conflicts and ruptures. In cases where
the terms of a monogamous relationship agreement have been violated, practitioners need to explore whether the agreement is meeting the needs of all partners,
whether the contract was consensual or coerced, and whether the rupture is due to
a values conflict between partners (e.g., autonomy norm vs. permission norm) or
due to the existing agreement not matching the desired arrangement.

Evaluating relationship quality

The contrast between actual evidence and commonly held assumptions in the
field of relationship counselling further demonstrates the need for practitioner
familiarity with relevant research findings. Although Cohen's (2016) experiment
on perceptions of relationship satisfaction among monogamous, open, and polyamorous "couples" [sic] found that monogamous couples were assumed to have
higher relationship satisfaction than "open couples", Muise et al.'s (2019) study
of 1,054 "consensually nonmonogamous" people found that people who were
more sexually fulfilled in their "primary" relationship also reported greater relationship satisfaction with their "secondary" partner. Similarly, in a study of 1,093
polyamorous people, Mitchell et al. (2014) found that participants with two con-
current romantic partners reported high levels of need fulfilment and satisfaction,
and there was no association between need fulfilment with one partner and relationship satisfaction with another.

Therapists often rely on mononormative biases when evaluating polyamorous
and multi-partnered relationships. Some couple-centric relationship quality indicators that are often applied to relationship counselling with polyamorous and
multi-partnered people include:

- The age of relationship initiation (e.g., "met and married at 18").
- The chronological duration of the relationship (e.g., "married for 20 years").
- Whether they are cohabiting.
- Whether they have procreated or are raising children together.
- Owning a home and/or other assets together.
- Formal relationship recognition, particularly marital status.

- Public and social recognition (including whether or not a particular partner has met their partner's biological parents, work colleagues, or members of their spiritual and cultural communities).
- Whether they are "sexual partners" (some polyamorous relationships are non-sexual).
- Whether they are *fluid bonded* (a term for people who do not use barriers to prevent bodily fluid exchange during physical intimacy).
- Whether they are a woman/man dyad.

These mononormative indicators have all been critiqued by polyamorous communities as biased and unhelpful (Kean, 2018; Klesse, 2006). For example, *comet* relationships, which have "elliptical orbits like comets in space" (Graham, 2019), challenge the mononormative assumption that the quantity and frequency of time spent together is a universal indicator of relationship quality. Comet relationships may be deep, spiritual connections with only infrequent contact due to geographical distance or existing capacities (see Ansara, 2020 to learn more about the existential and emotional significance of comet relationships).

In contrast to the aforementioned mononormative relationship indicators, Fern's (2020) *HEARTS of being secure* (HEARTS) model identifies "the different ingredients, skills, capacities and ways of being required for secure functioning in multiple attachment-based partnerships" (Fern, 2020, p. 173). Fern's model, which was developed through an evidence base of actual polyamorous and multi-partnered people, includes these polycule-centred indicators of relationship quality:

- Here (being here and present with me).
- Expressed delight.
- Attunement.
- Rituals and routines.
- Turning towards after conflict.
- Secure attachment with self.

Whereas couple-centric indicators focus primarily on external and societal markers to determine relationship quality, the polycule-centred HEARTS model indicators prioritise affective experience, interpersonal skills, personal development, and relational dynamics.

From default dyad thinking to polycule-centred practice

Polycule-centred practice requires a shift away from *default dyad thinking*, in which dyads are viewed as the "natural" base unit of relational systems. Polycule-centred therapists support therapy participants to examine their own mononormative biases and re-evaluate their perspectives, relationship agreements, and boundaries. Some key clinical elements of polycule-centred practice are:

- Investigating and acknowledging coercive/compulsory monogamy.
- Not assuming polyamory is inherently less consensual.
- Recognising polyamory is not necessarily "open".
- Being aware of the power and privilege dynamics when a relationship built as a "two-person tent" wants to "open up".
- Investigating apparent "infidelity", "affairs", and "cheating" in terms of whether the monogamy was with informed consent, coerced, compulsory, or a relationship agreement breach.
- Respecting and valuing the needs of everyone in the relational system.
- Identifying and addressing couple privilege, hierarchical privilege, and other mononormative biases.
- Making sure relationship configurations and agreements are negotiated and consensual, not "mono by default".
- Clarifying relational norms (i.e., autonomy vs. permission norm).
- Addressing relational ruptures that result from non-consensual hierarchies, compulsory and coerced monogamy, and changing awareness and needs.
- Engaging in psychoeducation so people are aware of diverse relational structures and norms.
- Helping people to identify and address privilege and bias in their relational system.
- Identifying non-consensual, mononormative relational dynamics such as:
  - Unicorns – People who join a dyad but are not consulted in relationship decisions.
  - Lassoers – "I'm your one true love! You know you only want me."
  - Love Police – "Do what you want *sexually*, but you can't *love* anyone else!" (In effect, the Love Police rule promotes the sexual objectification of other partners.)
  - Pyramids – "I have to matter the most!"
  - Islands – "I want nothing to do with your other partners!"

Although it is beyond the scope of this chapter to provide clinical guidance on how to address each of these common multi-partnered relational dynamics, practitioners can facilitate exploration in relationship therapy by using polycule-centred language like the terms I use earlier.

Conclusion

Mononormative biases are deeply entrenched in sex therapy and relationship counselling. This situation is improving as more polyamorous therapists and therapy participants challenge our erasure and marginalisation. Applying polycule-centred practice can strengthen people's relationships, improve their communications, and address their core emotional needs in a relational system in a more equitable and ethical way.

References

Anapol, D. (2010). *Polyamory in the 21st Century: Love and Intimacy with Multiple Partners*. Lanham, MD: Rowman & Littlefield Publishers.

Anderson, E. (2010). "At least with cheating, there is an attempt at monogamy": Cheating and monogamism among undergraduate heterosexual men. *Journal of Social and Personal Relationships*, *27*(7), 851–872. https://doi.org/10.1177/0265407510373908

Ansara, Y. G. (2020). Challenging everyday monogamism: Making the paradigm shift from couple-centric bias to polycule-centred practice in counselling and psychotherapy. *Psychotherapy and Counseling Journal of Australia*, *8*(2). https://pacja.org.au/2020/12/challenging-everyday-monogamism-making-the-paradigm-shift-from-couple-centric-bias-to-polycule-centred-practice-in-counselling-and-psychotherapy/

Barker, M. (2005). This is my partner, and this is my . . . partner's partner: Constructing a polyamorous identity in a monogamous world. *Journal of Constructivist Psychology*, *18*(1), 75–88. https://doi.org/10.1080/10720530590523107

Barker, M., & Langdridge, D. (2010). Whatever happened to non-monogamies? Critical reflections on recent research and theory. *Sexualities*, *13*(6), 748–772. https://doi.org/10.1177/1363460710384645

BBC News. (2012, August 28). *Three-Person Civil Union Sparks Controversy in Brazil*. Retrieved from www.bbc.com/news/world-latin-america-19402508

Benedict, L. A. (2017). *Polyandry Around the World*. Retrieved from http://digitalscholarship.unlv.edu/award/28

Brown, J. D. (2019). *Anti-oppressive Counseling and Psychotherapy: Action for Personal and Social Change*. New York: Routledge.

Cassidy, T., & Wong, G. (2018). Consensually nonmonogamous clients and the impact of mononormativity in therapy. *Canadian Journal of Counselling and Psychotherapy*, *52*(2).

Cohen, M. T. (2016). The perceived satisfaction derived from various relationship configurations. *Journal of Relationships Research*, *7*, E10. https://doi.org/10.1017/jrr.2016.12

Coyote. (2019, March 9). *A Genealogy of Queerplatonic*. Retrieved from https://theacetheist.wordpress.com/2019/03/09/a-genealogy-of-queerplatonic/

Creation, K. (2019). *This Heart Holds Many: My Life as the Nonbinary Millennial Child of a Polyamorous Family*. Portland, OR: Thorntree Press LLC.

Du, S. (2016). Gender norms among ethnic minorities: Beyond '(Han) Chinese patriarchy'. In X. Zang (Ed.), *Handbook on Ethnic Minorities in China* (pp. 240–262). Cheltenham: Edward Elgar Publishing.

Fern, J. (2020). *Polysecure: Attachment, Trauma and Consensual Nonmonogamy*. Portland, OR: Thorntree Press LLC.

Fox, J. C. (2020, July 1). Somerville recognizes polyamorous relationships in new domestic partnership ordinance. *Boston Globe*. Retrieved from www.bostonglobe.com/2020/07/01/metro/somerville-recognizes-polyamorous-relationships-new-domestic-partnership-ordinance/

Fricker, M. (2007). *Epistemic Injustice: Power and the Ethics of Knowing*. New York: Oxford University Press.

Girard, A., & Brownlee, A. (2015). Assessment guidelines and clinical implications for therapists working with couples in sexually open marriages. *Sexual and Relationship Therapy*, *30*(4), 462–474. https://doi.org/10.1080/14681994.2015.1028352

Graham, S. (2019, June 13). *The Joy of Comet Relationships – Part 1*. Retrieved from https://loveuncommon.com/2019/06/13/comet/

Grunt-Mejer, K., & Łyś, A. (2019). They must be sick: Consensual nonmonogamy through the eyes of psychotherapists. *Sexual and Relationship Therapy*, 1–24. https://doi.org/10.1080/14681994.2019.1670787

Harré, R., & Parrott, W. G. (Eds.). (1996). *The Emotions: Social, Cultural and Biological Dimensions*. London: Sage.

Haupert, M. L., Gesselman, A. N., Moors, A. C., Fisher, H. E., & Garcia, J. R. (2017). Prevalence of experiences with consensual nonmonogamous relationships: Findings from two national samples of single Americans. *Journal of Sex & Marital Therapy*, *43*(5), 424–440. https://doi.org/10.1080/0092623X.2016.1178675

Heckert, J. (2010). Love without borders? Intimacy, identity and the state of compulsory monogamy. In M. Barker & D. Langdridge (Eds.), *Understanding Non-Monogamies* (pp. 255–266). New York: Routledge.

Henrich, J., Boyd, R., & Richerson, P. J. (2012). The puzzle of monogamous marriage. *Philosophical Transactions of the Royal Society of London. Series B, Biological Sciences*, *367*(1589), 657–669. https://doi.org/10.1098/rstb.2011.0290

Henrich, R., & Trawinski, C. (2016). Social and therapeutic challenges facing polyamorous clients. *Sexual and Relationship Therapy*, *31*(3), 376–390. https://doi.org/10.1080/14681994.2016.1174331

Hua, C. (2001). *A Society without Husbands or Fathers: The Na of China*. New York: Zone Books.

Hyde, J. S. (2005). The gender similarities hypothesis. *American Psychologist*, *60*(6), 581–592. https://doi.org/10.1037/0003-066X.60.6.581

Jenkins, C., & Rickert, E. (2020, November 2). *Canada Defines Love – Exclusively*. Retrieved from https://ncsfreedom.org/2020/11/02/canada-defines-love-exclusively/

Jordan, L. S. (2018). "My mind kept creeping back . . . this relationship can't last": Developing self-awareness of monogamous bias. *Journal of Feminist Family Therapy*, *30*(2), 109–127. https://doi.org/10.1080/08952833.2018.1430459

Kaldera, R. (2005). *Pagan Polyamory: Becoming a Tribe of Hearts*. Woodbury, MN: Llewellyn Worldwide.

Kean, J. (2015). A stunning plurality: Unravelling hetero- and mononormativities through HBO's *Big Love*. *Sexualities*, *18*(5–6), 698–713. https://doi.org/10.1177/1363460714561718

Kean, J. (2018). Sex/love skirmishes: "swinging," "polyamory," and the politics of naming. *Feminist Media Studies*, *18*(3), 458–474. https://doi.org/10.1080/14680777.2017.1393760

Kipnis, L. (1998). Adultery. *Critical Inquiry*, *24*(2), 289–327. https://doi.org/10.1086/448876

Kisler, T., & Lock, L. (2019). Honoring the voices of polyamorous clients: Recommendations for couple and family therapists. *Journal of Feminist Family Therapy*, *31*(1), 40–58. https://doi.org/10.1080/08952833.2018.1561017

Klesse, C. (2006). Polyamory and its "others": Contesting the terms of non-monogamy. *Sexualities*, *9*(5), 565–583. https://doi.org/10.1177/1363460706069986

Klesse, C. (2011). Notions of love in polyamory – Elements in a discourse on multiple loving. *Laboratorium. Журнал социальных исследований*, *3*(2), 4–25.

Klesse, C. (2013). "Loving more than one": On the discourse of polyamory. In A. Jónasdót-
   tir & A. Ferguson (Eds.), *Love: A Question for Feminism in the Twenty-First Century*
   (pp. 77–90). London: Routledge.
Klesse, C. (2014a). Poly economics – capitalism, class, and polyamory. *International
   Journal of Politics, Culture, and Society, 27*(2), 203–220. https://doi.org/10.1007/
   s10767-013-9157-4
Klesse, C. (2014b). Polyamory: Intimate practice, identity or sexual orientation? *Sexualities, 17*(1–2), 81–99. https://doi.org/10.1177/1363460713511096
Klesse, C. (2016). Marriage, law and polyamory. Rebutting mononormativity with sexual
   orientation discourse? *Oñati Socio-Legal Series, 6*(6), 1348–1376.
Klesse, C. (2019). Polyamorous parenting: Stigma, social regulation, and queer
   bonds of resistance. *Sociological Research Online, 24*(4), 625–643. https://doi.org/
   10.1177/1360780418806902
Legros, D. (2014). *Mainstream polygamy: The non-marital child paradox in the West.* New
   York: Springer.
Manduley, A. (2015, September 1). *Stop Saying "Poly" When You Mean "Polyamorous".* Retrieved from http://aidamanduley.com/2015/09/01/stop-saying-poly-when-
   you-mean-polyamorous/
Marriage Equality USA. (n.d.). *Our Story.* Retrieved from www.marriageequality.org/
   about
Matsick, J. L., Conley, T. D., Ziegler, A., Moors, A. C., & Rubin, J. D. (2014). Love and
   sex: Polyamorous relationships are perceived more favourably than swinging and open
   relationships. *Psychology & Sexuality, 5*(4), 339–348. https://doi.org/10.1080/1941989
   9.2013.832934
McGoldrick, M., Gerson, R., & Petry, S. S. (2008). *Genograms: Assessment and Intervention* (3rd ed.). New York: W.W. Norton & Company.
Mitchell, M. E., Bartholomew, K., & Cobb, R. J. (2014). Need fulfillment in polyamorous
   relationships. *The Journal of Sex Research, 51*(3), 329–339. https://doi.org/10.1080/00
   224499.2012.742998
Mogilski, J. K., Reeve, S. D., Nicolas, S. C., Donaldson, S. H., Mitchell, V. E., & Welling,
   L. L. (2019). Jealousy, consent, and compersion within monogamous and consensually
   non-monogamous romantic relationships. *Archives of Sexual Behavior, 48*(6), 1811–
   1828. https://doi.org/10.1007/s10508-018-1286-4
Moors, A. C., Rubin, J. D., Matsick, J. L., Ziegler, A., & Conley, T. D. (2014). It's not just
   a gay male thing: Sexual minority women and men are equally attracted to consensual
   non-monogamy. *Journal für Psychologie, 22*, 1–13.
Muise, A., Laughton, A. K., Moors, A., & Impett, E. A. (2019). Sexual need fulfillment
   and satisfaction in consensually nonmonogamous relationships. *Journal of Social and
   Personal Relationships, 36*(7), 1917–1938. https://doi.org/10.1177/0265407518774638
Naftulin, J. (2019, November 16). *Being in an Open Relationship Isn't the Same as Being
   Polyamorous. A Sex Researcher Explains the Difference.* Retrieved from http://images.
   markets.businessinsider.com/difference-between-polyamory-open-relationships-
   swinging-2019-11
Nordgren, A. (2006). The short instructional manifesto for relationship anarchy. *The Anar-
   chist Library.* Retrieved from http://theanarchistlibrary.org/library/andie-nordgren-the-
   short-instructional-manifesto-for-relationship-anarchy.pdf
Pallotta-Chiarolli, M., Sheff, E., & Mountford, R. (2020). Polyamorous parenting in contemporary research: Developments and future directions. In A. E. Goldberg & K. R.
   Allen (Eds.), *LGBTQ-Parent Families* (pp. 171–183). Cham, Switzerland: Springer.

Pieper, M., & Bauer, R. (2005, November). *Mono-Normativity and Polyamory*. Paper presented at the International Conference on Polyamory and Mono-Normativity, University of Hamburg, Germany.

Ritchie, A., & Barker, M. (2006). "There aren't words for what we do or how we feel so we have to make them up": Constructing polyamorous languages in a culture of compulsory monogamy. *Sexualities, 9*(5), 584–601. https://doi.org/10.1177/1363460706069987

Robinson, M. (2013). Polyamory and monogamy as strategic identities. *Journal of Bisexuality, 13*(1), 21–38. https://doi.org/10.1080/15299716.2013.755731

Rubin, J. D., Moors, A. C., Matsick, J. L., Ziegler, A., & Conley, T. D. (2014). On the margins: Considering diversity among consensually non-monogamous relationships. *Journal für Psychologie, 22*(1), 19–37.

Sheff, E., & Hammers, C. (2011). The privilege of perversities: Race, class and education among polyamorists and kinksters. *Psychology & Sexuality, 2*(3), 198–223. https://doi.org/10.1080/19419899.2010.537674

Sheff, E., & Wolf, T. (2015). *Stories from the Polycule: Real Life in Polyamorous Families*. Portland, OR: Thorntree Press LLC.

Shih, C. K. (2000). Tisese, and its anthropological significance. Issues around the visiting sexual system among the Moso. *L'Homme,* 154–155, 697–712. https://doi.org/10.4000/lhomme.56

Tervalon, M., & Murray-García, J. (1998). Cultural humility versus cultural competence: A critical distinction in defining physician training outcomes in multicultural education. *Journal of Health Care for the Poor and Underserved, 9*(2), 117–125. https://doi.org/10.1353/hpu.2010.0233

Twist, M. L. C., Prouty, A. M., Haym, C., &, VandenBosch M. L. (2018). Monogamism measure. *Sexual and Relationship Therapy: International Perspectives on Theory, Research, and Practice, 33*(4), 376–381. https://doi.org/10.1080/14681994.2018.1526883

van Tol, R. (2017). I love you, and you, and you too: Challenges of consensual nonmonogamy in relationship therapy. *Transactional Analysis Journal, 47*(4), 276–293. https://doi.org/10.1057/9781137002785_8

Wilkinson, E. (2012). The romantic imaginary: Compulsory coupledom and single existence. In S. Hines & Y. Taylor (Eds.), *Sexualities: Past Reflections, Future Directions* (pp. 130–145). London: Palgrave Macmillan.

Wolf, T. (2013, August 31). *Polycule*. Retrieved from https://kimchicuddles.com/post/59867573481/polycule-you-can-always-keep-up-with-the-most

Wolf, T. (2015, May 27). *Polycule*. Retrieved from https://kimchicuddles.com/post/120040274525/sneak-peak-at-whats-to-come-for-character

Wolf, T. (2016, May 29). *Updated Polycule!* Retrieved from https://kimchicuddles.com/post/145121785030/updated-polycule-for-full-character

Zeitzen, M. K. (2020). *Polygamy: A Cross-cultural Analysis*. London: Routledge.

Chapter 2

Loving freedom (beyond monogamy – opening up a dyad)

Niki D

Introduction

In Western societies, a perception of monogamy as superior to consensually non-monogamous relationships still reigns supreme. In such a mononormative culture (Pieper & Bauer, 2006), relationship commitment and relationship health are judged as sexual and romantic exclusivity to one person at a time. The journey beyond this prescribed relationship model is likely to encounter prejudice, misunderstanding and condescension.

As psychotherapists, we are as seeped in dominant cultural and political values as our clients. These social contexts inform – and misinform – our beliefs, norms and standards of relationship ideals. Adopting a non-judgemental position on relationship diversity is the very least we can offer our clients. However, to genuinely support and understand clients in open and polyamorous relationships, we need an awareness of the variance of relationships that are not monogamous, as well as knowledge about the specific challenges and delights of our clients living and loving in such expansive ways. We may also be required to adapt existing narrow therapeutic frames in relationship therapy to meet the unique requirements of multi-partnered relationship constellations.

In this chapter, I focus on what a therapist needs to attend to in themselves – and in sessions – when individual clients or monogamous couples want to open up their relationship. I will make use of case examples to bring the dynamics of this complex relationship negotiation alive.

The co-creation of a unique non-mainstream relationship can be a wonderfully empowering and uniting experience for couples who have been an exclusive dyad. It can also be intense, exhausting, confusing and anxiety-provoking. Due to this complexity, I am introducing a 7-stage model to co-creating open relationships that I hope can offer a helpful structure for therapists and clients.

Privileging the pair – therapist bias

> We judge what we don't understand.
>
> (unknown source)

DOI: 10.4324/9781003260561-3

There is a mainstream assumption that monogamy is a relationship style that the majority of people are in, want to be in and want others to be in. Exceptions to this can be found in teenage and young adult sexual experiences, LGBTQ and BDSM communities and some faith-based cultures (Barker & Langdridge, 2010).

In fact, even referring to monogamy as a relationship style would confuse many. It suggests there is a choice, a negotiation, a contemplation about what is best for an individual going into a sexual/romantic relationship. Such a thought-through decision seems unthinkable to many. It demonstrates there are other options, it hints at fluidity, at variation to a relationship style norm that is rarely questioned. Yet questioning how and why we chose the relationships we are in is an important consideration.

Psychotherapy training and relationship therapy courses rarely discuss relationship diversity. To develop our knowledge around any non-mainstream subject, it is left for trainees and experienced therapists to find our own way to books such as this one.

My chapter does not promote one relationship style over another. Open or polyamorous relationships may suit people at some points in their life, with a particular person or people. Whilst monogamy might also suit them at other points. Conversely, there may be only one type of relationship which fits someone no matter who comes into their life, and holding onto this relationship style may be more important than adapting to the other person's needs.

What I want to promote is the freedom to question the norm and the robustness to challenge the 'norming' of relationship styles that most of us are embedded in.

We all hold biases, make assumptions, and have opinions that exclude others. The ethical consideration as therapists is how this might affect our work. Are there people we would not be able to work therapeutically and ethically with?

Although we cannot bracket all our biases, or even be aware of all our assumptions, we can commit to understanding what might act as a barrier to clients talking openly with us about the non-exclusive intimacy they bring into their world.

With this in mind, I want to talk briefly about identity labels.

Labels and language

Language is one way we have of obscuring or clarifying, including or excluding. As therapists, we aim to become attuned to the impact of our words, our speech patterns, our tone, and our silences.

I don't believe we all need to be using the same terminologies, have read key books, have lived in certain ways, or shared particular identities in order to work therapeutically and ethically with GSRD clients.

Certainly, having lived experience of being marginalised does offer us a mind/body felt knowledge of discrimination and oppression which our GSRD clients know all too well. However, the attitude we bring to our connections and conversations with clients can be far more important than shared experiences and identity.

I use the term 'open relationships' to refer to any relationship style that embraces sexual and/or romantic involvement with more than one person outside and/or within the dyad relationship. This may include people that define their open relationship styles as polyamorous, swinging, monogamish or casual.

I was convinced by Dr Y Gávriel Ansara's argument (Chapter 1) against using non-monogamy as a term due to its problematic binary reference. For those of us that opt for open and polyamorous relationships, being defined by what we are (open, polyamorous, swingers, relationship anarchists, etc), rather than what we are not (non-monogamous) is my preference.

When I say open relationship, I am typically referencing a dyad – a couple – who co-create their relationship connection in a way that allows for an openness (of an agreed extent) towards others and themselves. An openness to explore their sexuality, intellect, their bodies, emotions and their lives. These clients may use terms such as 'opening up our relationship', 'moving towards being polyamorous' and 'queering our dynamic'.

It is respectful to use whatever terms and identity labels our clients choose to describe themselves, rather than becoming rigid about terms which can prevent us from holding a therapeutic stance.

Relationship diverse clients report mainstream therapists as lacking knowledge of open relationships, feeling their relationship issues are marginalised and the therapist is biased against open and multi-partnered relationships (Heinrich & Trawinski, 2016). For example, equating multiple sexual partners with immaturity and fear of commitment, or expecting them to choose between partners (Orion, 2018).

In my practice, I have heard examples of previous therapists eroticising a client's polyamorous life and over-sharing their own desire to open their marriage and take casual lovers. Or of therapists assuming the problem in a client's relationship is down to it being polyamorous when this is not the case, or totally ignoring the open relationship as it was too far out of the therapist's comfort zone. My clients were left feeling fetishised or marginalised and certainly misunderstood.

Even the most aware and culturally competent of us need to continue educating ourselves and questioning our assumptions, never arriving at a self-satisfied full stop.

It can help to ask ourselves the following questions:

- What were the relationship models around me growing up?
- What was the type of relationship that was promoted as healthy and desirable in my culture?
- How did I see those types of relationships working out? What were the positives and the negatives for the people in those types of relationships?
- What did I hope for in sexual/romantic relationships as I became a teenager, a young adult? (if applicable)
- What kinds of messages about open relationships did I hear from those around me, both in society as a whole and the individuals in my life?
- Where did I see open relationships modelled, and what did I feel about them?
- What has informed my own views about closed and open relationships?

- What have the positives and negatives been for me about closed relationships (if any)?
- What have the positives and negatives been for me in open relationships (if any)?
- Do I believe that someone can love and/or be in love with more than one person at a time?
- How closely are sex and love linked for me, and what role does sex play in my relationships?
- Do I have different sexual fantasies, needs, desires than my partner/lover – and could we fulfill each other's sexual desires?
- In a world without judgement, what relationship style would I most enjoy? And why?
- What stops me from seeking out these relationships now? (if applicable)
- What are my judgements and/or cautions about closed and open relationships?
- If I feel my own relationship style choice is 'healthier' or 'superior' to other types, what am I elevating in myself, and what am I denigrating in others?
- Do I use the term 'couple therapy' in my advertising? If so, do I deliberately want to exclude multi-partnered relationships?

Whilst working on our own biases, let's also listen out for – and respectfully challenge – statements of monogamous supremacy or ignorance from other therapists, in peer supervision, from supervisors, teachers and colleagues.

We are in a socio-economic, political culture that pedestals human coupling. *Couple privilege* is a term used in polyamorous circles which highlights the advantages afforded two people who share a life together as primary partners and choose to prioritise their relationship over their connections with other lovers and/ or romantic relationships. There is no way of avoiding couple privilege. It is what people do with their privilege that matters most.

Mononormativity – client bias

> If you are always trying to be normal, you will never know how amazing you can be.
>
> (Maya Angelou)

Life is one big improvisation. We are all just making it up as we go along! Some people are anxious about this level of uncertainty, freedom and the responsibility that inevitably comes with it, so they rely on the dominant discourses of how 'to do' life. Others are more prepared to fly by the seat of their pants.

There is usually an implicit understanding between a couple of what monogamy means without any discussion ever taking place.

I have worked with couples where only one partner has a desire for an open relationship of some kind. Sometimes referred to as a hybrid relationship (Barker & Langdridge, 2010). An affair or another crisis in the relationship may have accelerated the need to address their relationship dynamics. Where there is a mono/poly mix in the relationship, there is inevitably work for therapists to do around spotting biases and assumptions at play.

It requires us to notice and point out any self-righteous language and attitudes that we may see in monogamous clients when their polyamorous lover/partner challenges them. If not, we run the risk of letting the monogamous client's indignation and shaming become oppressive and abusive in the session. As Taormino points out: "If you play by all the unspoken rules of monogamy when you are in your monogamous relationship, you learn some things you're going to have to unlearn"

(2008, p. 212).

Listen out for statements of mononormativity in comments such as the following:

> "I wouldn't risk my relationship for casual sex".
> "Our sexual life is sacred and I want to protect that, not water it down".
> "I need to be someone's first choice".
> "I thought I knew you, now it feels like I didn't know you at all".
> "You are enough for me, why can't I be enough for you?"
> "If you don't feel jealous/guilty then you can't really love me".
> "It's because you are bisexual/pansexual/trans that you want other lovers".
> "Can't I satisfy you sexually?"

Of course, it is equally possible for shaming statements to come from the partner who wants to open the relationship. It is as important to notice a client pushing their agenda of relationship openness when their monogamous partner is not ready or desiring of this relationship style.

How we challenge our clients' biases remains the same as challenging any other reductive way of thinking. A therapeutic challenge is always an invitation to see something differently – to pause and reflect on an opinion or decision that has not been examined previously.

For this reason, it is crucial that we have already worked on our own relationship biases so that we don't collude with one client's perspective and miss important comments that need to be clarified within the dyad.

Opening up a dyad – challenges and delights

> Sexuality can awaken us to our interrelated being. A way of knowing ourselves through someone else.

(Smith-Pickard, 2014, p. 84)

Clients intending on opening a closed relationship need to negotiate, communicate clearly, identify needs and desires, establish boundaries, bump up against them, and then re-clarify those boundaries once more. It is everything that occurs in a closed relationship but dialled up a notch and with a few extras thrown in.

While writing and reflecting on the people I have worked with, I realised there is often a cycle – a series of seven stages when evolving into an open relationship. Each stage is important, and has its own set of challenges. When a stage is skipped, I have inevitably found people struggling. I certainly know this myself when I have negotiated opening up monogamous relationships. For me, the learning was in the doing and then the undoing of things that did not work well.

There is no rigid formula to opening up a relationship. The stages I have identified may help guide people who are co-creating their new relationship together. My model can assist us as therapists become attuned to stages that clients seem to be missing or getting stuck in.

Every person, every dyad, every triad, quad, polyamorous family or group does it differently. However, there are tried and tested aspects of having an open relationship which are likely to lead to better outcomes.

7-stage model to co-creating an open relationship

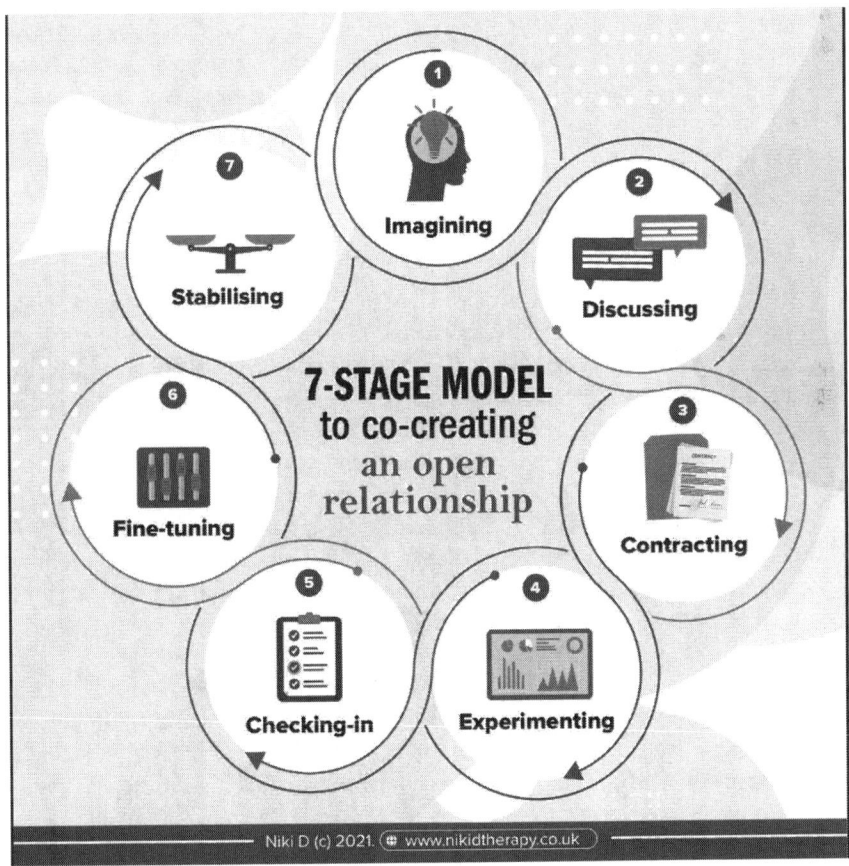

Figure 2.1 7-stage model to co-creating an open relationship.

Stage 1: Imagining

When you think outside the box there is more freedom to be creative, to tailor-make a relationship that moulds to your unique combination. Let your imagination wander, dream without judgements, enjoy playing with other possibilities in your mind. Take yourself and your partner seriously in your daydreaming but also have fun with it. Make it about you and your wishes, desires, hopes and needs. Without censoring, invent and create other worlds, other relationship scenarios.

From the expansive freedom of these ideas, start imagining what these scenarios might feel like in your life. For example, imagine how it would be to go on a date then return home to your partner, imagine it the other way around. Imagine having an exciting threesome and seeing your partner's arousal and pleasure with someone else. Imagine your partner seeing your sexual pleasure also. Picture falling in love with someone else or vice versa. Imagine you both fall for the same person or living in a triad, a quad. Envisage going to play parties, picture being the one who stays home. Picture your friends, family, colleagues, neighbours, unexpectedly seeing you kissing someone else. Visualise coming out to those groups of people. Keep going. Follow where your imagination takes you. Notice if you avoid thinking about certain inevitable aspects of being in an open relationship. Find the honesty within yourself to face this and identify what your resistance is about.

Stage 2: Discussing

Now is the time to pull your ideas out of the clouds and the rainbows and into the space between you and your partner. Start talking about it all and don't rush it. Do what you can to ameliorate any stress or pressure when discussing this topic. Decide on the attitude you want to take when you discuss it. Agree on pausing the conversation if it gets tough. Consider as a couple how you deal with differing opinions, disagreements and with conflict. Do you become adversarial? Does one of you sulk, become defensive or emotionally and physically withdraw? When conflict arises, how might you stay connected? Can you rise to the challenge of differing viewpoints and see it as an exciting aspect of your relationship dynamic that keeps you on your toes, intellectually, emotionally, politically?

Identifying and articulating your relational values is important. If you go off track, come back to your intention with your partner. What values are important to you both, and are you living them or not? Hold an attitude of curiosity about each other and the topics you are discussing.

Agree on a time frame. Notice each other as you talk. Observe each other's body language as much as what is said. This conversation is about something you will co-create, so you both need to talk, and you both need to listen well also. This type of discussion will interweave throughout the rest of your relationship together. The more sophisticated you get at communicating clearly and respectfully, the easier the process becomes.

Stage 3: Contracting

Out of dreaming and discussing comes decisions. If you continue to discuss and imagine and never live out any of your ideas, then work out what is going on. Is it safer to stay in this comfort zone? How you contract can be as varied as you both are. It can be written, verbal, drawn out in thought bubbles. The point of this stage is getting realistic, uniting in your decision, teasing out the grey areas and the sticking points. It is about clarifying expectations, conjecture and half-truths under the bright light of a relational conversation. Be real about the limitations you may need to face together. It is not a legal document; it is a focus for you both to come together and do the relational work in a deliberately thoughtful way. Ensure you attend to this stage when you are both calm and clear headed and feel emotionally open and connected to one another. This type of relational contracting is about respect, negotiation and clarification. It isn't about manipulation or dominance. Consider if you want to use veto power, no rules or somewhere in between. What will your hard boundaries be (limit situations) and soft boundaries (limits that can be negotiated)? Try and cover it all. Except of course you won't!

For more information on contracting, read Tristan Taormino *Opening Up* (2008). Or for therapists, Rhea Orion's *A Therapists Guide to Consensual Nonmonogamy* (2018).

For this to be effective, you will both need to be honest, even when that honesty conveys something your partner, or even you, might struggle with.

People can feel that having a contract offers something solid to hold onto. Yet you cannot contract out uncertainty. Everyone and every relationship pose the same risks. So, what you are actually committing to is uncertainty, but with some clear guidance to help pave your way over life's rocky ground.

Stage 4: Experimenting

Relationships are always an experiment, and now it is time to get out there and start experimenting. Go on that date, follow up that lead on Grindr, Feeld or OkCupid. Invite that gorgeous group of open-minded people you met recently to dinner. Check out a swingers, trans, BDSM or polyamorous event. But try something. Smaller steps might be the more prudent idea at first, but not always. Honour the limits you decided on in your contracting. There will be time to make changes to your agreement later. Most important is the respectful manner you continue to hold towards each another (and others of course).

Ask yourself what you want from this beginning stage. Are you wanting to plunge into a new world of sexual and relational possibilities with abandon or with caution? Do you want to commit yourself to new ways of connecting with others and not replicate old, unhelpful relational habits? Although this stage is about discovering more about yourself and new people, hold in mind what might be discovered about your existing relationship too. Your time, attention and energy need to be directed here also.

Be mindful of what I call the 3 D's: discomfort, disruption or damage. Situations which elicit discomfort might prove useful to stay with as you adapt to something new. Other scenarios may become disruptive to your life in ways that can be positive and transformative or be problematic and create damage. I recommend Jessica Fern's book *Polysecure* (2020) for clear guidance on addressing relational wounding and attachment panic. It is really important that you do not push yourself to adapt to a scenario which generates an emotional crisis and attachment trauma.

Stage 5: Checking-in

Do this often! It doesn't have to be a lengthy and serious review every time a new experience outside of your dyad takes place. However, there does need to be a 'how are you feeling about . . . ?' 'What was it like when this happened?', 'I would really like to talk to you about . . .'

There can also be more regular, quick check-ins when you notice you or your partner struggling. If the timing isn't right, let them know it is something to return to. If you find yourself swerving the check-ins, identify why and address it. Hold realistic expectations. Things will go wrong. There will be boundaries crossed, there will be poor communication, there will be other people's feelings and situations to factor in. You are likely to find out lots of useful information in this stage. Stay attuned to yourself and your partner as you talk. You might notice jealousy, anxiety and excitement. All these feelings offer you a guide towards what needs attention. If you feel insecure and uncomfortable with the level of sharing, or with certain activities or people involved, speak about this so you avoid acting it out instead. Identifying and then articulating your feelings is important, but so too is understanding what led to a particular emotional response. What is that emotion conveying? What needs to be either soothed or addressed in relation to how you are feeling? Is it ingrained socio-cultural messages that don't sit with your values and need to go? Is it an indicator that something is not right in your relationship dynamic? Or is it an emotional clue that a certain boundary is needed or that you want to slow the pace down?

Checking-in is a way of giving and receiving information so you can move into the next stage of this opening up process.

Stage 6: Fine-tuning

With the ongoing checking-in process, you both will have far more information and experience, more wisdom and humility, to fine-tune your open relationship and the peaks and dips along the way. This stage may involve going through the other five stages again, and again. It helps smooth off the rough edges in your relationship. It might mean you need to start therapy; or address a relational trauma you have avoided for years. It might mean coming out to others, changing your living situation, or a shift from sexual to non-sexual in an important relationship. It could mean tightening your safer-sex agreement, or loosening your veto powers. Your values and views may have changed. You certainly will have altered in ways that could be wanted or unwanted. In this stage you will need to tease out imbalances in your relationships, communication problems, sexual issues and emotional challenges like possessiveness, guilt, insecurity and neediness. This is the stage where you realise that equality in your relationship is not about perfect balance and symmetry. There will be an imbalance in an open relationship. One partner may be having a wonderful time with multiple lovers, whilst you are struggling to get some dates on the go. We all come in a context, and the factors of your context might mean there is a smaller pool of people to choose from.

Look for the information in your emotional reactions, and use it to make decisions that are healthier for you and your relationships. Look for where you feel a threat (perceived or actual) and where you find safety. This stage is not the time to hide in either naivety or cynicism. Both positions mean you are avoiding dealing with something important. Resist the urge to be self-critical or judgemental about the feelings you have. This is the stage for the development of emotional intelligence and emotional resilience.

Stage 7: Stabilising

You got there! Don't make this stage your aim, as you will miss out on some of the complexity and fun along the way. However, feel proud of yourself and your romantic and/or sexual others when you realise how steady and special your open relationship is. Because of course it won't always be, so enjoy the calm waters for now. Honour your personal growth and resilience, your capacity to 'walk your talk', and show integrity by living out your values in your relationships. Keep cherishing your relationships and yourself. Keep humble too – it is likely you will be plunged back to any of the other stages at some point.

Stabilising can also include a return to a closed relationship. In which case celebrate your courage for trying out something many people swerve and instead have non-consensual affairs. Celebrate your dignity in reaching limits in yourself and your relationships and deciding to accept these. Turning away from open and polyamorous relationships can also mean turning away from strongly held principles and a group or community that supported and encouraged you. Notice this, grieve this, and find allies.

Case examples – intersectionality and variation

> It's not about finding the right person; it's about being the right person.
>
> (Mary Pender Greene on Esther Perel networker master classes webinars)

To protect the identity of clients, I've used an amalgamation of client scenarios, and all identifying details have been altered. The situations described reflect the variance of contexts and responses that my clients have presented with.

Opening up a dyad for the first time

Meet Ash and Kai, both in their late twenties, living together for four years. Ash is British, with Irish/Jamaican heritage, and identified initially as trans masculine non-binary, but after top surgery started defining as a queer, trans man. Kai is British/East Asian, gender fluid and femme presenting. They are attracted to masculinity and reluctant to label themselves beyond that.

They are both strongly involved in the queer scene in their professional and personal lives. Monogamous relationships were rare in their social groups, and Kai had previously been in open relationships. Both felt ready to expand their relationship, or as Ash said: 'to queer our relationship'. He had been the one who raised it, as coming out as a trans man left him wanting to explore his body and sexuality with new partners, including more masculine presenting people. They both wanted to invest in opening up their dyad thoughtfully and carefully with the safety zone of therapy to hold them steady.

They came for short-term relationship therapy, contracting for twelve sessions, with the last six sessions paced out to a pattern that suited them at that stage.

The sessions with Kai and Ash moved at a fast pace due to their readiness for change and their knowledge of open relationships. They requested 'homework', so I sent them an adapted questionnaire from Dr Tammy Nelson's book *The New Monogamy* (2013). Nelson's questionnaire can help facilitate a discussion about what possible situations with others are acceptable or not to a couple.

By the second session, after they had written their own relationship contract, Kai and Ash wanted to talk about how to manage problems they could foresee when they started dating other people.

For this, I suggested the down to earth book by Tristan Taormino *Opening Up* (2008). They read it separately and highlighted parts to discuss in session three. They were a whirlwind of productivity! They also made use of Taormino's checklists of four categories to consider when designing their open relationship. The four W's (2008, pp. 122–135). **Who**: relates to new people's characteristics, familiarity, orientation. **What**: the types of connections, what activities are allowed and what boundaries are needed in relation to this. **When**: refers to logistics of time, frequency, duration. **Where**: the physical place, events allowed, public vs private.

By session four they had both been on dates, and at the start of the session, I checked in to see how they wanted to discuss their dates. What would be too much information? Too little? How did they feel about sharing these intimacies with me and with each other? They had already practised asking the other to pause if they felt emotionally overwhelmed or upset. They were determined not to override their emotional responses – but use them as information that they could tune into instead.

Kai's struggle was related to Ash's date being more 'successful' than theirs. Ash was clearly attracted to his date, and there had been flirty exchanges by text since. Kai realised they needed a boundary around Ash not getting into sexually charged texting at home. Kai knew when Ash was aroused and in these early days found this threatening. This opened up a rich conversation in the session about sexual desire, being desirable/desired and imbalance around this theme being an inevitable part of most relationships and open ones in particular.

We considered whether an erotic charge could be enjoyed between them rather than being distressing or secretive. We talked about erotic compersion and the possibilities of changing a threat into an enticement. Erotic compersion (Taormino, 2008) is feeling sexual arousal from your partner's pleasure in someone else; it is the opposite of erotic jealousy.

I was deliberately encouraging a playful, flirtier and more creative attitude towards this topic, and Ash and Kai took it up and made it theirs.

An area in our therapy work that remains taboo is working with the erotic (Darnell, 2021). Esther Perel on her various YouTube talks and podcasts highlights this also. Our own ease about sex and sexuality will promote more dialogue on these topics among our clients.

It is not about flirting with clients, or getting our own sexual or egoistic needs met through clients. Rather, it is about allowing our own sexual, sensual, erotic selves to be a part of us in sessions, rather than trying to present as if we never had an erotic/sexual life at all, for those of us that have.

This case example shows how stages two, three and four can progress quickly for some partners and still be very effective. As Ash and Kai were embedded in a culture of openness around relationship dynamics, stage one had elicited no shame or secrecy that required teasing out and understanding. My work with this couple focussed mostly on stages five and six. The checking-in and fine-tuning stages.

When we ended our work, Kai and Ash decided to keep the same time commitment they had made for sessions with me. After discussing together how they might use that hour each fortnight, they opted for having the first thirty minutes split into each person speaking without interruption for fifteen minutes each; the second thirty minutes to discover the theme or issue that came out of the monologues and work together to find a way forward on this.

Opening up a single partnered relationship a second time

Meet Raf and Lennox. Two cisgender men, both gay and married for eight years. They are in their late forties and living together with three adored dogs. Lennox is black British of Caribbean heritage, and Raf is white Scottish.

They had a friendship circle of other cisgender men who were in closed and open relationships. Lennox had wanted an open relationship for some time, whilst Raf absolutely did not. He had felt pressurised by Lennox into giving it a go, and they opened up their marriage three years ago for ten months. It was a total disaster. They both ended up hurt, and their relationship was on the brink of collapse. They went for relationship therapy at that time for six months, and they limped back to monogamy.

When they reached out to me, their relationship had recovered, and they were stable in their lives. They wanted to mend the pain of their first attempt at an open marriage, and Lennox wanted to see if they could ever try it again in a healthy way. Raf was cautious, but this time confident he would not agree to any unwanted changes.

As our work progressed, it became clear they had skipped most of the stages my model refers to. Lennox had managed half of stage one. He had imagined what he wanted from an open marriage, but he hadn't gone on to ground his imagination in reality by inventing scenarios he might find himself in. There had been minimal discussion and no contracting, checking-in or fine-tuning. No surprise they never got to a place of stability.

Session example

I invited Raf and Lennox to spend an uninterrupted twenty minutes each talking about what open relationships meant to them. This might be enough direction for some clients, but as Raf and Lennox had a tendency to privilege their intellect, I added another element to their descriptive task.

I asked them to talk from the perspectives of their head, heart and gut. In various spiritual, body based and psychotherapy approaches, they are referred to as the three wisdom centres. This exercise offered my clients a structure to help them get in contact with their thoughts and values about open relationships, then in touch with their heart-felt, emotion-based feelings and finally their embodied sense-based response to this topic. This exercise can also include how the different parts communicate with each other: which was more dominant, which contradicted another part, which part felt silenced or ignored. The following is an extract of how powerful this mode of descriptive whole-body enquiry was for the two men.

LENNOX: My heart and body are yearning to matter to others, to be seen. My relationship with you Raf and our dogs is like water in a desert. You know how emotionally distant my family was and how fucked up I was by the racism I experienced at school. I didn't relate to anyone and was so excluded and socially awkward that nobody came toward me. I had no deep friendship, no intimate connection until I met you. I feel like I have a vibrant soul inside me that wants to be noticed. I love being in this marriage with you. I want no other husband, no other man to nest with. My heart tells me that I love you and I love what we have made together. It also longs to know how I could be with other men. Particularly other black men. I want to have intimate connections with black men as a way of understanding myself more, to heal from the racism I went through and to know that I can matter to more than one person and that more than one person could matter to me.

RAF: My heart and gut cried out against opening our marriage, but I felt in order for you to have a meaningful life and for us to stay together this poly thing had to happen, even though I did not want it. So, my suffering had to be ignored – but in ignoring it I felt that I stopped existing. Better to have my relationship exist, than for me to exist, and I couldn't have both. I felt suicidal, emotionally chaotic. My new boyfriend became my life raft to hold onto when I felt like I was drowning. I feel so bad that I used him like that, he was my stand-in for when my marriage to you collapsed.

LENNOX: I saw your distress and I didn't know how to resolve it. I felt that the only way out was to keep going through with it. I felt humiliated as I had wanted the open relationship and yet less than a year later you had a long-term lover and other meaningful connections and I hadn't even had a successful date. Then you told me you didn't want to do this open relationship anymore and my sense of fairness was outraged. So, I couldn't just say ok, I felt I just needed to have this one experience of being with another man for the whole awful year not to have been a terrible mistake.

Later on, I ask Raf to use his head, heart and body to consider how he felt about an open relationship now. He said his head-based response was excited by the prospect of sexual and romantic adventure, but in his heart, he felt an immediate block, a wall of shame and fear.

> My heart cannot allow me to imagine wanting someone else as it feels I would be betraying Lennox, as if I would be saying to him, you are inadequate, not good enough. To want other experiences with other people feels like a criticism towards him.

He described it as having a polyamorous head, a fearful heart and a tired gut.

> I am overloaded, I give enough out in my work, my relationship, to my family and friends that the thought of adding other lovers to my plate feels exhausting and overwhelming.

They both needed to grieve and forgive themselves and each other. To understand and to gain perspective and to identify gently together what they wanted to protect in their relationship now, and what they wanted to create together and separately in their lives. This work in long term therapy is ongoing as they talk through their 'acquired' views about open and closed relationships. It is humbling to see how trust can be rebuilt, fears understood, and sparks found in the embers of past chaos and pain. This time with space to think and feel and make use of whole-body intelligence. Acceptance is the first stage towards change, and I was watching it become a platform for their transformation.

Opening up a dyad to welcome a third

Meet Alex and Luna. Alex is a straight, cisgender man in his fifties. Luna is a bisexual, cisgender woman in her thirties, both are white, with Alex being British and Luna being Spanish. They had lived together for nearly a decade and had two children together.

When they came for therapy, they were already extending their relationship. Flirting with others, making out with women and femme, non-binary people at parties in front of each other and with each other. They had recently both fallen for a cisgender woman (Sammi) and had been enjoying a deeply erotic and sexual time as a threesome. The emotional and sexual intensity of this exchange had gathered momentum quickly, and Sammi had become their favourite topic of conversation, both together and separately. As a feminist, Luna actively rejected monogamy due to its patriarchal roots, whilst Alex identified with anarchy and embraced the anti-establishment freedom of swinging and relationship anarchy. They felt optimistic and joyful as their relationship naturally evolved in response to meeting Sammi.

Some of what is known about triads or thruples is the likelihood that, at some point, one person is going to feel left out or put in the middle of a conflictual pair dynamic. There is much to attend to in a three. As a thruple told me recently, "we have to attend to four relationships, our three dyad relationships and our one triad relationship".

The sessions initially focussed on the significant positives in their relationship with Sammi. It had infused the sex life of Alex and Luna, and they felt waves of compersion, including erotic compersion, when they were together.

About six months into their new triangle relationship, tensions and stresses started to show. Sammi began seeing another person and had less free time as a result. In their excitement about their new triad relationship, Alex and Luna had become possessive of Sammi. She was 'their' lover, their 'special one'. It revealed how the triangle had actually been a couple with a lover, Sammi being more like their unicorn (stereotypically a bisexual female with a male/female couple in a relationship) than a thruple.

I suggested that they could invite Sammi to join them for some therapy sessions. We talked about how this might feel, for them and for her. I said Sammi was also welcome to have an individual online consultation or a full session with me to level out some imbalance. We discussed confidentiality, which I would hold for any session I had with Sammi, just as I would for Alex and Luna's sessions. In the end, Sammi was keen to have a joint session without seeing me first. She felt confident in Alex and Luna's appraisal of me. I noted this decision and was interested to see if it was reflective of how she made other decisions. Did trusting other people's judgements work out well for her or not?

The triad session seating was already considered by Luna, Alex and myself. I have a separate room for groups, and the L-shaped seating allowed the three clients to sit without any one person feeling excluded. Previously I have suggested people sit on the floor in a circle so that threes and small group constellations can all see each other.

Much came out of that initial triad meeting and the subsequent joint sessions. Sammi, Luna and Alex clarified a number of concerns, addressed assumptions made and fears held. At the end of each joint session, I left the room first, affording them some privacy to end their session with a hug, tears mopped up, or to leave individually.

This dyad and trio had previously jumped over stage three, five and six of my model (contracting, checking-in, fine-tuning). They had focussed on stages one and four (imagining and experimenting) without the stages that ground and clarify. In therapy these were the stages they now focussed on, as they all explored their tendencies to have fun without the slog of planning or preparing. This became an important part of their work, and I was able to make use of the way we discussed, experimented, contracted, checked-in and fine-tuned our own flexible session arrangements as a model of how to communicate effectively.

There can be a need to be adaptable when working as a relationship therapist with multi-partnered clients. Our clients may require solo sessions, couple sessions with primary partners, joint sessions with paramours or metamours, triad sessions or small group sessions where polyamorous groups and families are involved.

By adopting a flexible but consistent stance, the therapist can contract verbally and/or in writing to offer a mix of individual, diad and triad/quad sessions for the partners to make use of when required. This model of flexible relationship therapy can reflect a style of relationship expansiveness and allow the therapist to model how fluidity can be ethically responsive.

Conclusion – never assume anything!

> You only understand people if you feel them in yourself.
>
> (John Steinbeck)

In my practice with clients in multi-sexual and/or multi-partnered relationships, I have made many errors along the way. Some errors I have realised and been able to work with, other failings I may never learn about. There can be a valuable opportunity in showing our willingness to accept our faults, to apologise, to allow our clients to input and express how they feel about our fallibility. We could even find ourselves following my 7-stage model as we check-in, fine-tune and in doing so establish stability again. Until the next time!

One lesson that keeps being repeated in my life is that I should never assume anything. The variance in open relationship styles, along with the different meanings they hold for our clients, can never be underestimated. One therapeutic mode of holding an open mind and open heart so necessary in our work with clients is to adopt a stance of 'un-knowing' (Spinelli, 2007), a phenomenological attitude which Spinelli describes as:

> The attempt to 'un-know' suggests the therapist's willingness to explore the world of the client in a fashion that not only seeks to remain respectful of the client's unique worldview, but also to be receptive to the challenges to the therapist's own meaning and narrational biases and assumptions.
>
> (2007, p. 64)

Such a stance supports us staying welcoming of our clients' worlds, bracketing our own interpretations, prejudices and beliefs about what is best for our clients, and in so doing allowing us to know them for the unique people that they are.

References

Barker, M., & Langdridge, D. (Eds.). (2010). *Understanding Non-Monogamies*. New York and London: Routledge.

Darnell, C. (2021). Sexuality, sex therapy & somatics. In bed with the most likely bedfellows. So why aren't they? *Sexual and Relationship Therapy*, 1–14. http://doi.org/10.1080/14681994.2021.1882672

Fern, J. (2020). *Polysecure – Attachment, Trauma and Consensual Nonmonogamy*. Portland: Thorntree Press.

Heinrich, R., & Trawinski, C. (2016). Social and therapeutic challenges facing polyamorous clients. *Sexual and Relationship Therapy*, *31*(3), 376–390. http://doi.org/10.1080/14681994.2016.1174331

Nelson, T. (2013). *The New Monogamy: Redefining Your Relationship after Infidelity*. New York and London: New Harbinger Publications.

Orion, R. (2018). *A Therapists Guide to Consensual Nonmonogamy – Polyamory, Swinging and Open Marriage*. New York and Oxon: Routledge.

Pieper, M., & Bauer, R. (2006). *Polyamory and Mono-Normativity – Results of an Empirical Study of Non-monogamous Patterns of Intimacy*. Unpublished article.

Smith-Pickard, P. (2014). Sexuality and gender for mental health professionals. A practical guide. *Existential Analysis*, *25*(2). London.

Spinelli, E. (2007). *Practising Existential Psychotherapy – The Relational World*. London: Sage Publications Ltd.

Taormino, T. (2008). *Opening Up*. San Francisco: Cleis Press Inc.

Chapter 3

Common presenting issues in consensual non-monogamy

DK Green

Introduction

CNM (consensual non-monogamy) is showing up in the therapy room with greater prevalence than in previous years. Sheff (2020) summarises very well the study conducted by Haupert et al. (2017) to illustrate such prevalence:

> Research indicates that at least 20% (estimates range from a low of 21.2% to a high of 32%) of people have some lifetime experience with consensual nonmonogamy, and 4 to 5% are currently in CNM relationships. That means CNM is far more widespread than previously thought, and people in the US are thinking and talking about it a lot more than they used to. This influx of discussion and awareness of CNM can feel like pressure for the other approximately 80% who practice monogamy (usually serial monogamy), cheat, or remain single.

In this chapter, we will explore how best we can serve this complex collective of CNM communities as therapists, whilst unpacking our own systemic, structural, cultural, and familial biases and beliefs towards these practices.

There are many ways of practising CNM including RA (relationship anarchy), hierarchical, solo-polyamory, open relationship, and more. We will summarise unfamiliar language or CNM 'jargon' such as frubbly, compersion, metamours, NRE, polycule, and polyfidelity in order to better navigate this diversity of relationship structure within the therapeutic setting.

People who practise CNM relationships have been pathologised, demonised, and discriminated against. They have lost family, friends, jobs, careers, and even their children due to these 'non-conventional' relationship styles. In regard to hyper-vigilance, minority stress, and discrimination in society, they share much in common with other minority diversities such as LGBTQIA+ or kink.

This chapter will examine when and in what circumstances CNM may be healthy or unhealthy for our clients, how best we can help resolve the issues they present in therapy (such as jealousy, time management, conflict, negotiation and

DOI: 10.4324/9781003260561-4

agreement breaches, judgement and rejection by family/friends), and how to come from a place of non-judgement for a client's relationships.

We will critically examine a prevalent argument that CNM is somehow a more evolved/enlightened way of navigating relationships, whilst learning to hold the nuanced understanding that either CNM or monogamy may be a healthy choice for a client in a similar way as we can be 'wired' gay or straight.

There are vast numbers of people living perfectly happily within CNM relationships; indeed many consider CNM a part of their identity or orientation. Bear in mind that those without issues or struggles will be unlikely to enter our therapy rooms. We will consider whether CNM is even relevant to the presenting client's work, whether session length needs to be adjusted, who needs to be invited into the room, and other therapeutic practice issues.

As a starting point, we shall avoid the pathologising assumption that CNM is about coercion, abuse, power-over, commitment, or attachment issues, for example. It may or may not be; just as within a monogamous relationship.

As stated, there are myriad ways CNM is practised, and even *within* those communities there exists 'judgement' of other CNM practitioners' choices. As therapists it is crucial that we work with our own judgement to enable a safer space for our clients to disclose and discuss freely.

In order for some of the less familiar words and jargon used in this chapter to be understood or looked up as required, here is a glossary of commonly used terms within CNM.

CNM – glossary

- **CNM** (consensual non-monogamy), ENM (ethical non-monogamy), and polyamory are often used interchangeably. This is inaccurate as polyamory is only one form of CNM, and there are many other ways in which CNM can be practised. The debate between using CNM or ENM is ongoing within these communities; who and how do we determine or define what is consensual, or ethical? The former is debatable (e.g. CNC [consensual non-consent]), although consent is thankfully a very prevalent ongoing community dialogue, and the latter is subjective; e.g. non-monogamy may be consensual, yet not perceivable as ethical. Yet this is the language currently in use by CNM practitioners, so it shall be used here.
- **Polyam**: A shortened form of the word polyamory; 'poly' was previously in widespread use, but 'polyam' is now growing in popularity as the initial shortened form was deemed culturally insensitive to Polynesians.

Diversities of non-monogamy

- **Open relationships**: partners choose to engage in sexual and/or emotional non-exclusivity/non-monogamy, e.g. monogamish, threesomes, other unconnected partners, agreements such as one night of sexual freedom a year, swinging, etc.

- **Polyamory** (Sheff, 2012): a created word (conflating Greek and Latin) intending to mean 'many loves'. The belief is that people are able to love more than one person or partner, concurrently.
- **Polyfidelity**: a closed group practising CNM with each other only, often a triad, quad, V style, etc. This word, polyamory, and compersion were born of a CNM commune named Kerista in San Fransisco which existed between 1971–91 (Nichols, 2021, p. 279).
- **Monogamish**: a generally monogamous couple with structured agreements around what is and isn't ok around CNM, e.g. time frames (once a month), occurrences, etc.
- **KTP (Kitchen Table Polyamory)**: a particular style of polyamory wherein everyone talks openly to each other, agreements are made together, meta-mours are generally involved and connected in some way.
- **Solo-Polyamory**: based on self as the primary partner, building connections with no expectation or assumption of 'relationship escalator' (societally accepted relationship steps of dating, co-habiting, marriage, children).
- **V or Vee**: one person as the 'hinge' with two different partners, who are not in a relationship with each other but may be friends/close.
- **Parallel**: two relationships with one person, where the two don't interact and aren't connected.
- **Hierarchical polyamory**: wherein some relationships take priority over others, whether due to practical reasons (nesting [living together], child-rearing, marriage), relationship style (kink or D/s [dominance/submission]), chosen style (coupledom privilege), etc. Critics question the dynamics of privilege, power-over, and currently, this form is gaining negative judgement within some CNM circles; however – despite the criticisms having merit – it should also be pointed out that many are perfectly happy living within this form of CNM for themselves. For example, kink relationships, open marriages, or swingers. Mutuality, consensuality, and reciprocity are key markers for success. Language around partners is sometimes seen as primary, secondary, and tertiary.
- **RA (Relationship Anarchy)**: "Relationship anarchy (RA), and 'relationshipqueer', are words for relationship styles, which question the idea that romantic relationships should be privileged over other kinds of relationships – both culturally and in individuals' lives" (Barker, 2019, p. 53). This term is critical of hierarchical value systems that frequently prioritise sexual over non-sexual relationships or romantic over non-romantic, or even romantic over platonic. Focus is on each relationship being unique and evolving, developing or ending as required. The concept is that love is abundant and people can have multiple, differing, meaningful relationships, concurrently. Also specifically that no type or kind of love is bigger, better, more important, or prioritised above another; e.g. familial love, sexual, or romantic love, friendship, love for a partner, deep affection for a housemate, etc. Related in concept to but not the same as what was previously referred to as egalitarian polyamory, meaning not having a primary partner, all were equal.

- **Polygamy**: the practice of having multiple, usually married, partners, often from a religious or cultural standpoint. Polyandry (1 female partnered with multiple males) or more commonly polygyny (1 male partnered with multiple females).
- **FWB (friends with benefits)**: friendships wherein occasional or frequent sex occurs, usually within an enjoyable and boundaried agreement.
- **Swinging**: the practice – often in specific club events designed for the purpose (sometimes in the home) – of usually emotionally monogamous couples engaging in extradyadic sexual activity with other couples or singles.
- **Cheating**: non-consensual, non-monogamy, but I have included it here as arguably it is still a form of non-monogamy. Generally, it causes great harm and upset; and also occurs within agreed, negotiated, and boundaried CNM relationships, which can even – perhaps surprisingly – be experienced as *more* harmful.

Further CNM jargon

- **Polycule**: a relationship grouping, or a specifically mapped group of people in various intimate (emotionally and/or sexually) relationships with each other.
- **Meta (metamour)**: a person's partner's partner, e.g. a partner's girlfriend, husband, nesting partner, etc.
- **NP (nesting partner)**: a partner with whom a person resides, living together in a shared home.
- **Comet**: (relationship) an occasional play partner or lover, one who comes into and out of one's life, like a comet.
- **Polysaturation**: a person reaching a point where they are unable to contemplate beginning any (more) new or additional relationships, whether due to time management or emotional capacity, etc.
- **Polyaffective**: non-sexual, emotional connections between metamours, family, friends, where the connection occurs directly via a polyamorous relationship, e.g. a partner's grandparent is very fond of another partner's child, or a partner's friend becoming close to another partner's sister (Sheff, 2018).
- **Polysecure**: having a secure attachment with the self and others.
- **Mononormativity**: the attitudes, thoughts, feelings, and behaviours we are all subject to due to systemic, structural socialisation (family, peers, media, etc.). The concept is that if having one partner only is generally the accepted, normative expectation, then due to cognitive or unconscious bias, those with more than one partner are subjected to discrimination, rejection, exclusion, etc., via normative assumption.
- **LDR (long-distance relationship)**: people in a relationship who live far from each other geographically and maintain their relationship with visits, letters, and online.
- **Ambiamorous**: being equally comfortable with either monogamy or non-monogamy in relationships.

- **Compersion**: the feeling of joy at witnessing or hearing about a partner's happiness or fun with another person. Being happy because they are happy.
- **Frubbly**: a similar word for compersion; particularly happy feelings towards metamours.
- **Wibble**: having a psychological or emotional 'moment' of being insecure or concerned about something happening within your relationships, e.g. jealousy, or FOMO (fear of missing out), insecurity, or fear of loss.
- **NRE (new relationship energy)**: new relationships can bring immense joy and excitement, the thrill is visible and can potentially create discomfort for pre-existing relationships. Can also create compersion.
- **Veto (power of)**: when one partner can say no to their partner being with another person or expect a partner to end or not pursue another relationship, usually a specific person, or particular act.
- **Unicorn**: usually (not always) bisexual and AFAB (assigned female at birth), in a relationship with a couple.
- **Unicorn hunters**: couples seeking a unicorn; ethically complex and difficult. (Potentially problematic examples: a person being treated essentially as a sex toy rather than a whole person with their own needs and wants; prioritising 'couples' privilege'; insisting the unicorn must be in a relationship with both people in the couple; a couple trying to improve an already ailing relationship can result in the unicorn being blamed, rejected, and hurt.)
- **OPP (one penis policy)**: when a couple agrees to one partner (usually the woman) dating a woman, but not another man. This is problematic (though still practised by many) due to the mistaken concept that sex with another woman is somehow 'not real sex' therefore somehow ok; it's misogynistic at the root.

Social context

When working with CNM clients, we must take into consideration the wider context; how it is to *be* (or practise) CNM, within the constraints of our current society. Unpacking the social, structural, systemic values and judgements (which pathologise and presume harm from the very concept and practice of CNM) can have beneficial results when working with a client's own internalised guilt, shame, and internalised mono-normativity. Psychoeducation in the client room around the influence of socialisation can help them to heal their internalised shame, with recognition of those internal dialogues around stepping outside of societal 'norms'. Be mindful that whilst bringing the client's awareness to socialisation and internalised negative bias, we should avoid demonising the results; we still feel how we feel, and that's also valid.

Our *relationship* socialisation dictates that we find a partner ('other half'), fall in love, marry, have children, and live happily ever after. The inferences of this normative relationship assumption are that they are (a) different, binary genders and (b) a couple, i.e. only two people in a relationship. This socialisation is further solidified with strong messages around possessiveness, jealousy, 'one true love', 'I should be enough', 'soul mates', etc., leading to the assumption that if you require or desire more than one partner, the problem lies with you. This 'traditional' social-isation is consistently and stringently impressed upon us throughout our lives via family, school, peers, colleagues, and the media. Interestingly this is historically a relatively recent development. As Barker (2019, p. 11) states, "The idea of forming a lifelong monogamous bond with one person on the basis of romantic love and sexual attraction really only came into its current form in the 1950s."

Even with a measure of progress being made regarding discrimination against sexuality and gender diversities over recent decades (same-sex marriage; 2013 UK, transgender rights; 2010 Equality Act, Gender Recognition Act, 2004, etc.), CNM still invites – more often than not – a substantial or even a visceral reaction, from those outside of CNM communities ("oh no, I could never do that").

CNM is *not* a legally protected status, unlike being trans or gay. You can still lose your job for being non-monogamous, and courts can use it against you in child residency (custody) proceedings.

Also bear in mind that despite the not insubstantial statistics mentioned at the very beginning of this chapter illustrating the numbers of those who *do* engage in CNM, that still leaves 80% of people who do not and likely never will. Potential reasons for not wishing to engage with CNM vary from the result of socialisa-tion whether consciously or unconsciously, a personal history involving infidelity (e.g. cheating father), jealousy/territorial (don't like to share), or simply personal orientation.

From over 6,000 clinical hours of private psychotherapy practice, it has become increasingly arguable that monogamy and CNM are simply parts of another spectrum of sexuality wherein one might be considered monogamous or non-monogamous by nature (though it is still problematic trying to remove the effects of socialisation from that theory). However, many people currently engag-ing in CNM *do* consider it to be a fundamental part of their identity, an orientation in itself, if you will, and clearly self-identify as such; which implies of course that monogamy could also be. More research is much needed within this area to clarify; though literal proof may be as yet unachievable, general consensus may be achieved, such as with gay and straight, or with transgender and cisgender. Similar research around kink to determine whether choice/preference or identity/ orientation may be required.

> Although polyamorous and kinky identities are distinct, the populations prac-tising them share such a variety of traits and considerable overlap in member-ship that they warrant joint analysis.
>
> (Sheff & Hammers, 2011, p. 201)

One thing is clear, whether it is by orientation or by conscious choice, how we show up for our clients as therapists when navigating these CNM waters is abso-lutely crucial.

Therapist considerations

As already suggested, our first task as therapists is to unpack our *own* socialisation, unconscious bias, and judgement, in order to be best positioned to serve clients coming into our therapy rooms from CNM communities. This would naturally include our own familial and personal experience, as well as the wider context of socialisation including media influence. Here are some further considerations.

Pathologising and discrimination

The pathologising and discrimination of CNM clients are unfortunately prolific, not only in the wider context of society. Many clients of diversity enter the therapy room with tales of previous negative and damaging therapy experiences. Some negative assumptions spoken to CNM clients, heard many times first-hand within clinical practice are that 'being non-monogamous is clearly the root of their issues', that the client 'being non-monogamous must be about attachment or commitment issues' (this has been widely debunked, e.g. [Orion, 2018, p. 23], [Fern, 2020, pp. 25–28]), that 'non-monogamy is clearly coercion or abuse'. Comments (judgements, thoughts, and beliefs) like these are pathologising and harmful to clients who already face such negative discriminatory and derogatory remarks in their daily lives, within families, and out in the wider world. They confirm pre-existing hyper-vigilance of judgement and, particularly coming from a therapist, do so much harm in validating – from a position of presumed authority – negative self-beliefs and internalised societal judgement ('polyphobia') within a specific therapeutic context which is intended to be healing and helpful. Do no harm is still the first rule of therapy.

Even if as a therapist one understands the context of and around CNM and is intellectually robust in working with it, personal opinion and judgement can and will still be felt and present in the room with a client. We must *do the work* to ensure that not only do we understand intellectually but that we understand and have a genuine felt sense of non-judgement around CNM. Constructive conversations with actual CNM practitioners may aid this; a growing theme among many diverse communities (of gender, sexuality, or relationship) is 'don't talk about us, talk to us'. Intellectual understanding can potentially expand to genuine affirmative attitudes, with experience witnessing positive personal stories and visible examples of CNM not being harmful, but proactively good, healthy, and beneficial.

Bear in mind that CNM practitioners who are busily enjoying life and having no issues will be very unlikely to appear in our therapy rooms; so it behoves us as developing therapists to seek out those communities to find those stories for ourselves. It can be easy to develop the belief that CNM impacts negatively upon its practitioners if all we are seeing is those coming into therapy with their struggles.

It can also be easy to fall into the trap of believing that the initial core trainings and aims of becoming therapists include the concepts of non-judgement, unconditional positive regard, and beneficence; therefore, if we approach all clients with this, that should be sufficient. However, unconscious bias is named unconscious for good reason; we are not *aware* of our blind spots, and often unaware of how deeply socialisation impacts upon *all* of us, in many contexts and on many subjects. Acknowledging and understanding those biases allows us to work on them; indeed the vast multiplicity and intersectionality of discriminations extant within our current society (race, sexuality, gender, disability, neurodiversity, age, etc.) means it is absolutely *essential* that we work on them. One accidental look of surprise or a disapproving glance from the therapist is a microaggression that can and will be perceived and felt as judgement, and can only be further harmful to our clients.

Practical considerations

• Firstly consider the following question: does the work required by the client have anything to do with their being non-monogamous? Often clients come to therapy with needs around other topics: childhood trauma, bereavement, grief and loss, anger management, etc. They may not wish to discuss their CNM with you at all; it may be irrelevant and if so only in the surrounding context, rather than it being related to their presenting issues. If so, do not enquire further into their CNM practices, either out of curiosity or to potentially find a problem; trust that if it *is* relevant, they will bring it to you when (*and only if*) they feel it is safe to do so.

• Do not expect your clients to educate you. They are investing in your time; educate yourself, on your own time.

• Consider the timings of sessions. If it is more than one person coming to you for therapy (couples or moresomes [multiple partner relationship]), you may need additional time for the assessment so that everyone has a suitable opportunity to speak and to allow for additional intake forms for example. If it's a multiple-partner polycule coming together, might your regular sessions also need to be longer?

• Who is attending or needs to attend? Is it one person who is coming for other issues, who just happens to be CNM? Is it one person who specifically *does* wish to discuss their CNM relationship/s? Or is it relationship (rather than 'couples') therapy, whereby other parties also need to attend? Do they all actually need to attend? As a therapist are you willing to see multiple clients in relationships together? Do you need to consider an upper limit on how many people you have the capability to work with together in one session, or does it become 'group therapy', and are you ok with that?

I have found that asking a client to answer these questions during the assessment is helpful; they will clarify what they're seeking from you, and you can negotiate these terms within your competencies.

Presenting issues

Wherein, we explore how we can best help our clients to resolve the specific consensual non-monogamy issues, with which they present (illustrated with composite case examples).

Jealousy

By far the most common issue that shows up around CNM in my therapy room is *jealousy*, likely the predominant reason (as well as socialisation) for the 80% who never engage with non-monogamy. Jealousy shows up as a territorial nature or via socialised conditioning, that of simply not wanting to share. Perhaps trust or insecurity is the issue, maybe reluctant or coercive sharing in childhood simply opens wounds on this topic in adulthood. Retaining objectivity is key here; as a therapist, we frequently hear only one side of the story. Sometimes a client is looking to the therapist for a 'reality check', i.e. 'am I reasonable in feeling jealous about this?' Unless you have a full relationship history and an excellent understanding of the dynamics, boundaries, and agreements involved, err on the side of caution; there may be good, honest intent on both parts. Don't presume through social conditioning that yes, 'this is bad', and 'you're right to be jealous'. You may do harm to an evolving relationship, with your good intent to empathise with your client, and that insidious socialised bias.

It is arguable that jealousy is metaphorically the 'vestigial tail' of human emotions. Certainly once upon a time, claiming and holding onto your mate was a matter of procreation and survival; but with the population as it stands now the question arises, do we really need it? Some CNM practitioners state that they don't feel jealousy at all, that it simply doesn't occur for them, or if so only very specifically and rarely. That said, jealousy is a very real emotion and can be felt deeply and viscerally, and have repercussions on wellbeing and mental health, and negative relationship repercussions around trust and safety. Your jealous client needs empathy and kindness and not for the therapist to climb into a negative hole with them.

Rhea Orion (2018, pp. 65–66) suggests the following techniques to help clients navigate jealousy: to learn thought-stopping, positive self-talk, calming, and communication skills to accept rather than avoid jealousy, self-soothe, and learn positive ways to share feelings and reconnect with each partner.

Remember also that there are many ways of practising non-monogamy; if the jealousy cannot be worked through in one CNM scenario, perhaps it can be with another? Remember also that CNM is simply not right for everyone. This can also prove to be the outcome of therapy on occasion; but do not presume it to automatically be the case, simply because someone is struggling to navigate it at that time. All relationships have those struggles and moments. Successful and happy CNM practitioners often have stories to tell about times when they had struggles.

Case study 1

A previously monogamous couple presented for therapy, seeking help to move towards an open relationship, was struggling immensely with jealousy (both). What they were aiming for was for an additional someone (or more) to be in complementary relationships with. Working through what the jealousy was representing for each, and how it was showing up for them, it transpired that it was the pain of breaking the emotional monogamy in relationship or 'love' terms that were the fundamental issue. When we worked through what they each really desired, it was exploratory additional sex, so we investigated swinging, or shared experiences, as a potential alternative. They successfully maintained the emotional monogamy they both wanted, whilst injecting levity and sexual fun into their lives, with other consenting adults seeking similar.

Case study 2

A CNM V thruple (threesome) presented for therapy with person A struggling with jealousy around client B (the hinge partner) and client C. They had all been working with this themselves for some months but were struggling to navigate it and feared for the relationship enough to seek help. In working with the person struggling, initially (as agreed) individually, the pattern of when the jealousy arose and 'what it looked like' for them showed that it was fundamental insecurity around being somehow less important than client C, to client B. Time wasn't being well managed by client B, and visible displays of affection were being hidden (to protect client A from feelings of jealousy). Client A had a general feeling of being excluded and/or deceived (hidden affection between B and C) and feeling less important to B due to their time management. Working again together with all three, they were able to discover the reassurance that radical honesty and open communication gave client A, B learned to manage the diary better to provide more equitable time for each, and B and C became less afraid of sharing intimate or affectionate moments in the same space; as Client A also learned to communicate openly and honestly when there were any issues. Within a few months all three clients were far happier generally, and the jealousy issues for the most part were entirely resolved.

Time management

As shown in case study 2, diary management is a common issue for many CNM practitioners; making time for multiple relationships is a real consideration. Spreading themselves thinly across work, family commitments, and multiple relationships can create a pressured and stressful situation, rather than one that brings happiness to all concerned. Polysaturation can occur, whereby an actively non-monogamous person recognises or accepts that they literally don't have enough hours in the day to engage with all the relationships that they might *like* to; leading to a 'maximum number' of relationships capacity. For a client this is a useful self-awareness, leading to less pressure, as well as less chance for others to be unintentionally hurt for lack of their time and attention.

As a therapist, do not seek a perceived 'best practice' number for relationships. CNM clients will vary widely in how much resilience and capacity for multiple relationships they have and how resourced they are to contain them; from just two to several. In the case of RA (relationship anarchy) practitioners, this number could indeed be many more, as they often can and do include all their sexual, romantic, friendship, important people/relationships of other kinds, without delineating or valuing some types of relationship over others.

There is within CNM communities an 'inside joke' (usually emitted amidst light-hearted groans) around partners sharing and being ruled by their Google calendars; for very good reason. This is often a great suggestion for those struggling to manage or juggle multiple relationships, creating transparency for all involved that can ease insecurities around 'why am I not seeing partner X enough', as well as being a practical strategy for finding times where partners are available. Equity of time spent with each relationship is *not* necessarily the aim, however; there may be, for example, a nesting partner who naturally physically sees the resident partner more, but has fewer date nights to enjoy outside the home than another partner. This might lead them to feel that their 'joy time' with the NP is far less equitable than another partner who sees their NP only once a week, but for date nights and fun only.

Negotiations and agreements

CNM couples/moresomes may come to you – a CNM knowledgeable professional – for help in setting up their relationship agreements and boundaries; to help them negotiate these things. As a therapist, you will need to do some background research on what these may look like.

They may also enter therapy to heal ruptures within the relationship when those boundaries or agreements are breached. As in any relationship, whether monogamous or non-monogamous, breaches of trust or broken agreements can cause irreparable damage. They do happen, however, and within CNM practitioners the answer isn't automatically – as so often in socially mononormative relationships – to simply end the relationship. CNM practitioners care a great deal about communication, as it is only with *excellent* communication skills that such multiplicity of relationships are possible. Navigating family, friends, partners, work, schools, etc. all take learning good communication skills, which are essential when you are living within any form of GSRD (gender, sex, relationship diversity). We are all human and do make mistakes, and CNM people are no exception.

Trust is easy to break and very hard to regain; but *not* impossible. Working with your clients it is crucial that you provide a 'safe enough' space for them to work through such breaches and loss of trust with each other. Be with the clients where they are at, and do not allow unconscious bias to influence your thoughts around what is right or wrong for them; let them work it through together and decide for themselves. Ask questions and gently challenge to invite their perspectives, signpost to reading materials, or engage in psychoeducation where helpful. But the autonomy of their CNM relationship choice must remain firmly with the clients.

Case study 3

A self-identified queer couple presented for therapy, both having additional relationships, deeply in conflict due to a breach of their relationship agreement. Client A had overstepped a current boundary (sexually with Client C), and Client B was clearly distraught and uncertain about continuing the relationship. What transpired through having a safe enough space that both of them could talk freely about this breach of trust was that Client A had in fact stuck to the 'letter of the law' rather than the 'spirit of the law', utilising the very words of the agreement to find 'wriggle room' in order to transgress it. This was clearly not ideal, and both disrespected and harmed client B and the relationship. Within sessions, Client A admitted and owned that this was unacceptable and regrettable, a violation and breach with damaging consequences. With much reparative conversation, clearly revised agreements, and a promise to 'not be an idiot again; they were able to choose to continue the relationship. Client B felt heard, seen, and understood. Client A was openly regretful and ashamed but was able to communicate clearly with sincere and reparative apologies to Client B, so the relationship continued. They reported back sometime later that, in fact, the experience had strengthened their close bond, finding they were far more honest with each other since the experience of opening up to each other in therapy.

Further presenting issues

The unhappy partner

A frequent appearance in the therapy room is that of 'the unhappy partner'. In working with the client/s the reason will make itself known. It may transpire that there is some level of coercion, potential abuse (e.g. cheating being justified as CNM, i.e. with no agreements), jealousy beyond an individual's capacity or resilience, or simply that there is a relationship style disparity and the unhappy partner is monogamous. Explore all possibilities before making the latter assumption; though it does transpire in some cases.

Unpicking whether CNM is healthy or unhealthy for the client/s

This will show itself within therapy sessions. If a client is fundamentally monogamous, then a CNM relationship will ultimately not be workable. Sometimes mental health considerations mean it may not be a viable choice (rejection sensitivity, emotional dysregulation, etc.). If there are general relationship issues such as communication, boundary, disparity of desire, then these things can often be worked through in therapy so long as the therapist maintains an open mind and an anti-oppressive and non-discriminatory stance.

Solo-polyamorist

Sometimes an individual comes to therapy to explore CNM for themselves, or to work through struggles with CNM while practising it. Simply remaining objective and open, exploring the different types to find the right fit, or working through what struggles they are having is sufficient. The key again is non-judgement of their choices and respect for their autonomy.

CNM couples or moresomes working through relationship issues

Work with as you would any relationship; there are simply more people in the picture to consider. As with any relationship therapy, sometimes clients can work through their difficulties together and reach a better working understanding of how to better navigate the relationship, and sometimes they cannot. The therapist's role is to witness, observe, and assist where able, not to judge or assume.

Religious or cultural disparity

People are individuals and as such can have disparities regarding faith, religion, or cultural differences; sometimes this comes up in the therapy room as causing relationship issues. Without a good working knowledge of different cultures and faiths, and how they view CNM, the therapist can choose to either (a) refer to a therapist working with that skillset or (b) provide as safe a space as possible for the client/s to work through these issues. Note: well-intentioned but uninformed therapists can – as all therapists can – intentionally or unintentionally subject clients to micro-aggressions, potentially rupturing the therapeutic relationship, requiring a great deal of work to repair. The former is the *safer* choice; specialist help is preferable to well-meaning but uninformed. If the therapist chooses to work with these clients, then further training on how to take ownership and make reparation for micro-aggressions and heal ruptures in relationships is particularly wise, including when working with clients of any type of diversity.

Couples wanting to open up their relationship (see Chapter 2)

First, investigate the current relationship: are they secure? How do they negotiate agreements? Are there extant relationship issues?, and so on. Much like the idea of having a child to fix an unhealthy or dwindling relationship, entering into the complex and challenging world of non-monogamy will not heal or fix a relationship, and will almost certainly end in disaster. Facilitate the couple exploring the different options of CNM to help them find the right fit, assuming the relationship is currently solid. Suggest they retain a CNM competent therapist whilst they explore, learn, and potentially run into difficulties.

Coercion, abuse, power-over

Elements of this may or may not enter the therapy room, just as there can be within any monogamous relationship. Dialogues may exist around pressure to engage in CNM, such as 'if you loved me enough', 'this is what's wrong/ it'll fix us' are unacceptable and abusive forms of coercion, and depending on the power dynamic within the relationship, potentially abuse of power-over. Another theoretical and emotion-laden argument sometimes levied for non-monogamy is that CNM is somehow a more evolved form of relationship, a higher consciousness attitude, of elevated spirituality, more self-developed or self-aware. Clinical experience has shown many instances where this argument or belief leads to an unwilling partner agreeing to something they are not in full consensual agreement with. It is false and untrue; monogamy along with any form of CNM are equally valid choices, particularly if we consider them as a part of orientation or identity.

External presenting issues

Sometimes simply bringing the client's awareness to these external issues, along with psychoeducation on their effects, can be a healing therapeutic tool.

Minority stress

A direct consequence of stepping away from socialised relationship assumptions, whilst still having to live in a mono-normative society that is systemically discriminating against you. Meyer (2003, p. 51) states that the additive effects of minority stress create discrepancies in mental health outcomes leading to disproportional levels of mental illness in marginalised groups.

Judgement or rejection by family and/or friends

This is a strong minority stressor. One of the key factors for mental health in any area of GSRD diversity is family support; it is a predictor of resilience and well-being. Rejection or abandonment by family is particularly detrimental. Therapy can be helpful in one of two ways (depending on client's choice): by helping the client to come to terms with the loss and rejection, or by developing good communication and boundaries skills so that the situation can be addressed, and potentially resolved.

Hyper-vigilance and discrimination

Created within the wider social context. Repeated experiences of discrimination evolve into a person being hyper-vigilant; they become extra aware, on alert, and sensitive to discrimination, with a consistent expectation of poor treatment.

Historical\family\systemic issues

For example, a family history of infidelity, knowledge of the pain and harm caused, leading to self-doubt, internalised mononormativity, guilt, and shame.

Relationship escalator issues

Another problematic socialisation is the expectation that relationships must take a timely and predetermined order of steps (escalator metaphor; Gahran, 2017, p. 19): dating, getting serious, commitment, co-habitation, family. Stepping off from that escalator is complex and difficult when pitted against these assumptions, both internalised and external pressure from well-meaning friends and relatives. One client may wish to pursue these steps whilst others do not. Even within CNM those hetero and mono-normative assumptions can persist and may require careful working with.

Personality clashes between metamours

Do not just assume it is harmful or abusive because the relationship looks different from a monogamous one, or from how you might expect it to look. Particularly and especially if the CNM relationship is within a kink context and involves consensual power dynamics (see also Dr Lori Beth Bisbey's Chapter 9 in *Erotically Queer*); it is vital that you self-educate on kink dynamics if this is an unknown area to you, as it is also prevalent with a not insignificant crossover with CNM communities.

Additional considerations

One of the key aspects of any GSRD diversity is the concept of community. If biological family rejects you, chosen family – 'people like me' – can serve as a familial support network. A familiar expression amongst GSRD clients is 'queer fam' aka queer family, which rather illustrates this point.

It is worth noting however that as is the case within many GSRD communities, there is also *intra-community judgement* and criticism; so that even within CNM practitioners' own communities there can be uniquely additional stressors and a felt lack of safety. For example, RA practitioners are generally critical of Hierarchical Polyam, polyamorous people can be dismissive of swingers as 'not polyam', and a V relationship, triad, or someone seeking one may *look like* a

Unicorn Hunters plus Unicorn, which often receives harsh criticism. It should be noted that ALL of these forms of relationship are perfectly valid when fully consensual, well informed, and causing no harm to anyone within the relationship. People will habitually judge and criticise each other; therapists should not.

Mostly CNM practitioners simply wish to go about their business, living life to the full, achieving successful relationships and lives, like any monogamous person. As Rubel and Bogaert (2015, p. 977) state, "Generally, consensual nonmonogamists report high levels of relationship satisfaction and happiness or levels that are at least on par with those reported by monogamists."

A CNM or polyamorous person does not have to be *in a relationship* to identify as CNM by nature or choice, e.g. if you're gay, you're still gay even if you're single.

CNM isn't only about sexual or romantic partners; asexual, aromantic, and demisexual people can be non-monogamous or polyamorous too.

Intersectionality – race, class, culture, gender, disability, neurodiversity, mental/physical health, kink – are all prevalent crossovers with CNM. Each factor of a client's diversity compounds minority stress, hyper-vigilance, discrimination, and oppression (it is cumulative). We cannot discuss one without recognising the vast Venn diagram of all other oppressed diversities. That said, the majority (certainly not all) of CNM practitioners are privileged, white, middle class, educated, and professional.

Conclusion and questions

Can we as therapists provide a safer, non-judgemental, collaborative, and affirmative space for CNM clients to explore their issues whilst being fully cognisant of our own feelings, thoughts, and beliefs around CNM? Does the therapist need personal CNM experience in order to be fully congruent with these clients, and if not, can they educate themselves well enough to achieve competency? Can we as therapists recognise our own limitations in terms of areas of competence, and refer on when necessary?

As therapists it behoves us and indeed is absolutely crucial that we work through our own unconscious biases and socialised judgements around consensual non-monogamy, to enable a safer space for our clients to disclose and discuss their CNM and issues with us freely and to work with them from an affirmative perspective. Recognise that just as we are all unique individuals, so are CNM practitioners with their own ways of practising CNM, their own autonomy and choices in life, and that they are entitled to our fullest understanding, compassion, and unconditional positive regard.

References

Barker, M.-J. (2017–19). *Gender, Sexual, and Relationship Diversity (GSRD), Good Practice across the Counselling Professions 001, BACP*. Lutterworth: British Association for Counselling and Psychotherapy.

Fern, J. (2020). *Polysecure, Attachment, Trauma and Consensual Nonmonogamy*. Portland, OR: Thorntree Press.

Gahran, A. (2017). *Stepping Off the Relationship Escalator*. Boulder: Off the Escalator Enterprises LLC.

Haupert, M. L., Gesselman, A. N., Moors, A. C., Fisher, H. E., & Garcia, J. R. (2017). Prevalence of experiences with consensual nonmonogamous relationships: Findings from two national samples of single Americans. *Journal of Sex and Marital Therapy*, *43*(5), 424–440. http://doi.org/10.1080/0092623X.2016.1178675

Meyer, I. (2003). Minority stress and mental health in Gay Men. *Journal of Health and Social Behaviour. American Sociological Association*, *26*, 38–56. http://doi.org/10.2307/2137286

Nichols, M. (2021). *The Modern Clinician's Guide to Working with LGBTQ+ Clients, The Inclusive Psychotherapist*. New York and Oxon: Routledge, Taylor & Francis Group.

Orion, R. (2018). *A Therapist's Guide to Consensual Nonmonogamy, Polyamory, Swinging and Open Marriage*. New York and Oxon: Routledge, Taylor & Francis Group.

Rubel, A. N., & Bogaert, A. F. (2015). Consensual nonmonogamy: Psychological well-being and relationship quality correlates. *The Journal of Sex Research*, *52*(9), 961–982. http://doi.org/10.1080/00224499.2014.942722

Sheff, E. (2012). *Evolution of the Term Polyamory*. Retrieved from https://elisabethsheff.com/2012/10/08/evolution-of-the-term-polyamory/

Sheff, E. (2018). *Relationship Anarchy, Polyaffectivity, and Chosen Families*. Retrieved from www.psychologytoday.com/gb/blog/the-polyamorists-next-door/201809/relationship-anarchy-polyaffectivity-and-chosen-families

Sheff, E. (2020). When consensual non-monogamy won't work for monogamous folks. *Psychology Today*. Retrieved from www.psychologytoday.com/us/blog/the-polyamorists-next-door/202002/when-consensual-non-monogamy-wont-work-monogamous-folks

Sheff, E., & Hammers, C. (2011). The privilege of perversities: Race, class and education among polyamorists and kinksters. *Psychology & Sexuality*, *2*(3), 198–223. http://doi.org/10.1080/19419899.2010.537674

Chapter 4

When sex, health and stigma collide

Counselling people who sex work (and their partners)

Cyndi Darnell

When you think of a sex worker, what imagery comes to mind?

Likely that of a woman, perhaps a trans woman, perhaps a woman of colour, standing on a street corner. Short skirt, red lipstick, long boots, leopard-print jacket, leaning into a car window. Her life depleted. Her individuality obsolete.

This image is one of stigma. Embedded into our collective mind as a stand-in for sex workers the world over. Their inner worlds, relationships, multiple intersecting identities, complexity and humanity are erased by the mere fact that they *work*. Selling sex renders them public property, reduced to a symbol of desperation and poverty without agency or respect. Sadly, this positioning, often employed and perpetuated by the very organisations allegedly there to help and support them, maintains the stigma around the labour of sex workers globally.

Sex work is considered *dangerous* not because of the work, but because it rejects, challenges and truly fucks with the social order of things (Matos & Haze, 2019; Rayson & Alba, 2019). Especially things like sex, power, women, gender and freedom; ideas most societies are still struggling to come to terms with both legally and ethically. By contrast, the dangerous work of fire-fighting, preserving law and order or serving in the military is considered *noble* – while sex work is perceived as dangerous because it's unsettling; not for the workers, but for the people around them. Many people care *less* for the treatment of people *doing* sex work while on the job than they care about their own discomfort in the presence of sex workers (Grant, 2014). It's not the work itself but this stigma that is most likely why sex workers will seek professional support for their relationships, mental health and overall wellbeing (Bloomquist & Sprankle, 2019).

This chapter will address sex work stigma head-on and provide clinicians with a fresh, honest and useful perspective on sex work and working with sex workers (and their partners) as clients. I'll offer suggestions on how to provide a truly affirming therapy practice for sex workers in both mental health and intimate relationships contexts that go beyond pleasantries and lip service of support. When we can truly see the individuals sitting in our practice for the unique humans they are – not just because of their work, but in spite of it – we are better able to provide a service that is as affirming as it is helpful.

DOI: 10.4324/9781003260561-5

What is sex work and who are sex workers?

The truth is sex workers are everywhere. Our numbers are immeasurable because our work is mostly discrete and underground, but not because we necessarily like it that way. We are of many genders, of many ages, races, ethnicities, abilities, orientations and classes (Pedersen et al., 2019; Goldenberg et al., 2021). Some of us are living with HIV, and others have experienced incarceration and/or have complex immigration histories (Goldenberg et al., 2021). We use the term 'sex work' rather than 'prostitute' as it better covers the myriad professions under the umbrella of sex work, highlights that sex work is in fact 'work' (Rule & Twinley, 2021) and because it has a less pejorative tone than terms of times gone by. Some of us hold PhDs, while others barely finished primary school but we rely on sex work for our living nonetheless. We work (or once worked) selling sexual services that may or may not involve explicit erotic touch, but certainly involve prioritising the erotic wellbeing of others as perhaps part of, or even all of, our income stream.

Our work and lives are fuelled by myths and untruths that further ostracise us and contribute to the social stigma that can be both debilitating and deadly. Such myths include the following:

- That our work is dangerous.
- That we are vectors of disease.
- That we are all drug-addicted.
- That sex work is all we can do.
- That criminalisation of either the sex workers or the clients is the only way forward.
- That choosing sex work is neither feminist, nor empowering, nor even a choice.
- That we are only doing sex work because of some profound, traumatic, childhood wound.
- That our work is not real work, it's easy money.

(Sawicki et al., 2019; Bloomquist & Sprankle, 2019)

Our labour includes traditional full-service work independently or as part of an agency, brothel-based work, street-based work, escorting, hand-relief, erotic massage, Sexological Bodyworkers, sexual surrogacy, sacred intimates, stripping, lap-dancing, tantrikas (Tantric sex providers), professional kink and BDSM practitioners, porn performers, web-camming, phone sex providers (Pedersen et al., 2019, Sawicki et al., 2019) and most recently running *Only Fans* accounts, while often simultaneously studying, being parents, running small businesses, supporting families and communities, or doing other odd jobs to supplement our incomes or simply live our best lives. While not everyone who works in these fields would call themselves *sex workers*, the work itself is a form of sex work, and may or may not be met with varying degrees of stigma and/or regulation control.

We are, just like other service workers, service providers. Some days our work is great. Other days it's awful. Yet our work is deemed dangerous, lowly and exploitative – not because of *what* we actually do, but because of *how we are imagined* and treated by the public (Grant, 2014). The social perception of our work and our lives renders many sex-worker exclusionary radical feminists (SWERFs), anti-sex work humanitarians, and occasionally our clients to see us as lacking dignity because of how our work makes *them* feel. Unlike wait staff, cab drivers and sandwich-makers whose work is equally unglamorous, their work does not upset the status quo thus protecting them from 'rescue' narratives via well-meaning but delusional SWERF activists.

Sex work as it is used within this chapter refers strictly and solely to *consensual adult sex work*, not the heinous crime of human/child trafficking (which affects many industries globally, including building construction and clothing manufacture), nor the highly problematic "non-consensual sex work" (CDC, 2019) used by trusted organisations like the Center for Disease Control though in our vernacular is called rape and sexual assault. This distinction between actual sex work and workplace rape and abuse is very rarely made clear within research, policy, the media or broader society. This further complicates the lives of sex workers because laws and policies designed to regulate human trafficking and sexual assault do not distinguish between consensual adult sexual activity and "force, fraud or coercion" (U.S Department of State, 2004).

I myself am a former sex worker, now with the privileges that a robust multi-degreed and credentialled education offer me. I am humbled to be presenting this chapter through the lens of being both a former sex worker and an established clinician, helping us understand why reducing stigma, shame and blame for sex workers is more than a good idea, but a core human right.

Stigma and minority stress

While a sexual minority status is typically assigned to lesbian, gay, and bisexual people, van Anders's (2015) sexual configurations theory defines a sexual minority as "a marginalized sexual social location in a power hierarchy that can refer to individuals or groups" (p. 1186). Applying this framework, sex workers are allied with the sexual minority population, and thus, clinicians will benefit from adopting and adapting sexual minority and GSRD literature when exploring approaches to working with sex workers and their partners.

Overwhelmingly, the work of sex work is *not* the work itself, but the stigma, discrimination and conditions sex workers must face in order to simply exist and do their work (Treloar et al., 2021; Grant, 2014; Matos & Haze, 2019; Bloomquist & Sprankle, 2019). Stigma in this context can be defined as "an attribute that is deeply discrediting" (Goffman, 1963, p. 3) and one that "turns someone from a whole and usual person to a tainted, discounted one" (Goffman, 1963, p. 3). What is crucial here, like with all sexual minorities, is how the focus on *individual attributes* suggests that the stigmatised individual is simultaneously the location *and* the source of stigma, rather than acknowledging how social, economic and political power inform the expression of stigma (Treloar et al., 2021).

Compared to workers in other service professions, sex workers experience much higher levels of stigma and discrimination (Benoit et al., 2015) from the public, institutions and mental health professionals. Furthermore, the constant call to show oneself as empowered produces a further effect of a victim class (Grant, 2014, p. 94) and adds additional labour to an already emotionally and psychically demanding job, overlooking that job satisfaction and empowerment are issues in many professions, including writing, education and academia. More recently, the impact of COVID-19 has taken a toll on many in-person service providers globally with increases in police brutality, loss of income and an inability to access economic support because their work is criminalised; not to mention the impact on migrant workers who face further discrimination for fear of reporting stigma and violence should their migration status be affected (Goldenberg et al., 2021).

Historically sex work and mental health research in academia have been complicated. Early literature cited a prevalence among sex workers of post-traumatic stress disorder, childhood sexual abuse and experiences of threats and sexual assault prompting a 'desire to escape' (Farley & Barkan, 1998). Pathologising narratives linking sex work to drug use, childhood trauma and HIV transmission are woven into research related to this population (Vanwesenbeek, 2001). The early studies, just like with kink and queerness across the board including same-sex attraction, gender dysphoria, fetishism, etc., attempted to draw a causal link between sex work, trauma and abuse, suggesting that people engage in sex work *because* they are damaged or abused. This research failed to acknowledge its own biases and shortcomings, and instead privileged 'deviant' narratives, removing the context and the humanity from the workers entirely. The idea remains for many that sex work *itself* is inherently violent and traumatic (Dworkin, 1981) rather than the impact of society's judgement and exclusion on sex workers' lives.

The assumption is that the prevalence of abused women in sex work (in contrast with the world at large where studies have not been undertaken to determine how many 'abused women' are attracted to professions like banking, hospitality, law, gardening or psychotherapy) is related to *the work*, rather than a consequence of living in a violent society that perceives misogyny and gendered violence as inevitable. This also informs why there is little research on the intersectional experiences of sex work, like how one's race informs and affects sex work stigma, and mostly excludes representations of male, transgender, non-binary and other intersecting identities experiences of sex work beyond that of solely cis-women (Sawicki et al., 2019; Geymonat et al., 2021). Furthermore, relying on historical data on sex work and sex work research is unreliable at best and biased at worst due to the omnipresent stigma that interferes with understanding the nature of sex work. We are wise to remain critical of research on sex work when the researchers or presenters have limited or no experience of sex work themselves. Sex work research has historically done little to examine and explore the contexts and limitations of its own research (Seib et al., 2009), such as the physical, psychic and legal environments that sex workers must endure (Geymonat et al., 2021). Nor has there been an abundance of researchers stemming from sex work themselves – typically academics and clinicians seeking a pathology within a profession they do not understand nor respect (Rayson & Alba, 2019). Furthermore, one of the most overlooked elements of the work of sex work is that in most parts of the world, sex work in many forms is criminalised and/or heavily regulated (Harcourt et al., 2010; Geymonat et al., 2021). The fallout of this is a significant and over-whelming contributor to the statistically poor mental health and well-being of sex workers (Sawicki et al., 2019, Rule & Twinley, 2021, Treloar et al., 2021). There can be severe legal penalties for engaging in sexual services as a business transac-tion (remember until very recently, sex for '*free*' was seen as a woman's duty), while regulation imposes tight controls on the business elements of sex work such as mandatory registration, limitations on the freedom of movement between cities and countries, forced and coercive sexual health testing (Scarlet Alliance, 1999; Geymonat et al., 2021) and in some parts of the world forced sterilisation (Center for Health and Gender Equity, 2016). Both criminalisation and regulation contrib-ute to reduced social status and poorer health due to increased third-party powers, including discrimination and police corruption, immigration control not to men-tion problems with financial, legal, government and political institutions (Rayson & Alba, 2019; Geymonat et al., 2021). Making up for gaps in one's resume where sex work was the sole job, or producing financial records in order to secure hous-ing, credit or a mortgage is fraught for sex workers, if not impossible. The push by many pro-sex work peer-support organisations and human rights committees recognise that full decriminalisation in contrast with mere legalisation not only transfers power to the hands of the workers themselves, but also prevents sex work from being driven underground, causing further harm to workers, their fami-lies, their clients and communities (Geymonat et al., 2021). Without full legal pro-tection, experiences of exploitation, abuse and violence from police, clients and other parties may not be taken seriously and investigated, while sex workers may avoid reporting violence for fear that they themselves will be charged (Shannon & Csete, 2010; Rhodes et al., 2008).

Stigma and mental health

The relationship between stigma and mental health is complex and still not fully realised. While sex work stigma is rife, not all sex workers feel its effects equally, just like not all sex workers experience debilitating mental health issues (Rayson & Alba, 2019). Broadly speaking, stigma is a major determinant of population health linked to stress, self-esteem difficulties, depression and suicidality (Ray-son & Alba, 2019), while sex work stigma itself can interfere with sex workers' willingness to access mental health services when they fear mandatory report-ing, discrimination and pathologisation by professionals ill-equipped to serve them without causing further harm (Bloomquist & Sprankle, 2019; Rayson & Alba, 2019; Sawicki et al., 2019; Treloar et al., 2021). Furthermore, stigma can contribute to stress, a reduction of self-esteem, and reduced or non-existent social support. One study of 30 independent female sex workers within a major U.S. city (Koken, 2012) found experiences and fear of stigma to be a core experience of many sex workers. Some additionally noted associated feelings of shame, and others noted the constant degree of vigilance required added to weariness and stress (Koken, 2012). Another study of brothel workers in Sydney, Australia (Donovan et al., 2012), where sex work is decriminalised, showed sex workers enjoyed levels of mental health that were comparable to the general population. However, it's been suggested that while decriminalisation is an excellent first step, social stigma still impacts many workers in a variety of ways (Treloar et al., 2021).

Additionally, workers who are parents face further complications with the threat of their children being harmed because of their work stigma or removed by authorities should the parent be 'found out' sex working (Dickson, 2019). Others again report complex and unstable intimate partnerships (Johnson, 2019; Matos & Haze, 2019) due to the misconceptions around their work and dealing with partners' jealousies and discomforts in a world where sex is misunderstood, relationships skills are considered 'soft-skills', and sex work is a crime.

Benefits of sex work

While much is written on the shortcomings of sex work, there are also a variety of benefits to the work that many sex workers find affirming and encouraging (Antebi-Gruszka et al., 2019; Bloomquist & Sprankle, 2019; Grant, 2014; Pedersen et al., 2019; Treloar et al., 2021). These include the following:

- Being able to manage one's own hours offers flexibility, especially to those with complex family responsibilities.
- Being one's own boss and in control of one's own finances boost confidence and job satisfaction.
- A useful job for people living with inconsistent mental health as choosing one's own hours reduces the fear of a boss firing them for not turning up to work.
- Opportunities to practise setting boundaries and professional negotiation.
- Increased sexual health awareness.
- Affirming one's confidence through validation from clients and other sex workers.
- Shared support into creating and cultivating resilience and self-care to maintain physical and mental health both on and off the clock.
- The opportunity to earn a significant income (under the right circumstances).

Later in this chapter, we will also discover the most effective recorded mental health and emotional supports sex workers have devised for themselves and their communities, highlighting resilience in the face of stigma as a core component of community strength and wellbeing.

Guidelines and exploration for better practice

This section of the chapter will outline some useful sex worker–specific affirmative guidelines for clinicians to increase their competence in working with this community both individually and in couple's therapy/coaching contexts.

Sex workers seeking support from clinicians and social workers will be reaching out for a variety of reasons, many of which have nothing to do with the machinations of their work, but a lot due to the stigma, discrimination and complexity of their job when both on and off the clock (Bloomquist & Sprankle, 2019). While counselling sex workers and their partners does require a unique set of knowledge to offer truly affirmative care, the skills developed by clinicians and health care workers already working with other marginalised and stigmatised groups can hone their skills in working with minority stress theory alongside affirmative therapy guidelines for other members of the GSRD community already impacted by a variety of stigmas and discrimination.

Just as LGBTIQA+ individuals' general wellbeing reflects the way in which stigma, internalised homophobia, identity concealment and disclosure are managed (Hatzenbuehler, 2009), sex workers also struggle with stigma management, internalised '*whorephobia*' (the practice of internalising shame and stigma due to one's professional identity or practice – in this case, a direct result of sex work stigma) and worker concealment and disclosure issues related to their work (Koken, 2012). Therapists who are competent in sex worker affirmative therapy acknowledge first and foremost the impact of sex work stigma, in contrast to assuming distress is caused solely by the work itself (Benoit et al., 2018). This is the core guideline for working with both individuals and couples borrowed from 'gay affirmative therapy' (Langdridge, 2007) that goes beyond simply acknowledging that gay people should be treated with the same respect as heterosexual people as a bare minimum of ethical practice, but instead strongly affirms the client's identity and experience with the goal of reducing the harmful effects of sex work stigma and internalised 'whorephobia'.

Clinician's professional development and education

Getting educated is crucial to working with diverse populations, and sex workers are no different. While it's acceptable for practitioners to ask clients about unfamiliar terms, promoting oneself as 'sex worker affirming' means taking on an additional level of education to understand issues faced by sex workers in your specific location and their specific context, including understanding how local law impacts sex work, their clients and lives. While opportunities for CPD/CEs in this area are infrequent (Pink Therapy offers one), there are an increasing number of resources created by sex workers and sex work adjacent communities designed to assist with stigma reduction (Jeffreys, 2009; Bloomquist & Sprankle, 2019; Treloar et al., 2021). While good intentions matter, it's crucial we recognise that not all education is equal, and we must check sources of knowledge before deciding if the education offered is truly sex work affirming, or has its roots in 'rescue' narratives that serve only to further marginalise and harm sex workers by tricking them out of their jobs and shaming them for doing this work. If attending presentations at conferences it can be helpful to enquire:

- Does the presenter have a history of sex work?
- If not, have they collaborated with current or former sex workers for this presentation?
- Was the study and research developed with the needs and care of sex workers top of mind?

(Bloomquist & Sprankle, 2019)

Using these points helps to determine if the content is truly sex worker affirming. Beyond this, there are a variety of sex work educators to follow on social media along with publications written by current and former sex workers (see Appendix 4.1).

Furthermore, making connections with the sex worker community can be useful, but one is cautioned to tread gently and not step in to disrupt or interfere in marginalized spaces without having a sex worker background. Such organisations include the following:

- NSWP: Global Network of Sex Work Projects.
- Sex Work Hive (UK).
- National Ugly Mugs (UK).
- African Sex Workers Alliance.
- PROUD Nederland.
- Scarlet Alliance (Australia).
- Putas Feministas (Argentina).
- Sex Workers Outreach Project (SWOP) (USA).
- PACE Society (Canada).
- NZPC Aotearoa New Zealand Sex Workers' Collective (New Zealand).

Creating inroads within these communities serves to increase practitioner competence in their relevant regional context and establish trust with the workers and community at large. Many of these organisations maintain a list of trusted *sex worker friendly* professionals from therapists and medical professionals (like those listed on Pineapple Support: https://pineapplesupport.org/) to accountants and hairdressers that one can apply to be listed on.

The slogan "Nothing about us without us" is often used in sex work literature and peer education to reinforce the idea that knowledge relating to the work of sex work can only be shared, disseminated and used as educational materials when sex worker involvement is prioritised and assured. Using this ethos as a guide will enable you to discern helpful sex work training, as opposed to stigmatising and shame-inducing training from non-government and other not-for-profit organisations whose existence and funding rely exclusively on pulling consenting adult sex workers out of their jobs, and placing them in lower paid labour, all in the name of so-called 'liberation'.

Create visibility of your affirming practice

Just as LGBTIQA+, kink and polyamory affirming therapists will display a variety of rainbow/trans/BLM affirming stickers, flags, and statements around their offices, websites or social media, offering the same signalling to sex workers (the red umbrella is the symbol for sex-work worldwide) invites them to see you as a trusted source who is not only aware, but affirming. Remember sex workers may not disclose their sex work status to you initially or at all, and they may also not refer to their work as 'sex work' while still feeling the brunt of social and psychic stigma, minority stress and discrimination. To practise affirming support, the focus remains on how the client experiences the contexts of their work, rather than encouraging them to leave their work as the sole option to end their 'problems' (Antebi-Gruszka et al., 2019; Bloomquist & Sprankle, 2019). It also takes the position that sex work is indeed viable, worthy and valid. Unless the worker speaks of wanting to find different employment for *their own reasons*, as clinicians we do not attempt to redirect or 'rescue' them from their work.

While our intake forms may ask about clients' histories, it's important to note that there can be significant distrust of authority, including health and medical workers, from sex workers, especially working in locations where sex work is criminalised and/or where mandatory reporting is required. This can make intake forms asking about sex worker disclosure (Antebi-Gruszka et al., 2019) a thorny issue for both clinicians and sex workers. While some suggest asking about sex work from the outset is an affirming practice, it is not necessarily the best practice option in all circumstances. Discretion is advised.

Managing enquiries and guiding discussions

As with all counselling, the qualities of empathy, congruence and unconditional positive regard are crucial to sex workers too. Furthermore, it's been suggested that clients benefit when we mirror the language they use to discuss and describe their work (Antebi-Gruszka et al., 2019; Pedersen et al., 2019) rather than sanitising or altering it. Avoid questions that delve into their experiences of sex work that you may find titillating, fascinating or intriguing (Treloar et al., 2021; Antebi-Gruszka et al., 2019), but do nothing to thicken the story of the sex workers' reasons for seeking support. Examples like asking about *their* clients, asking about activities on the job and other such information are irrelevant unless the sex worker–client specifically brings them up as a source of distress. Remember that sex workers seeking support are unlikely to need support *for their job*, but more likely are seeking resources to support them in their personal lives to manage the feelings of shame, discrimination and inadequacy imposed upon them.

Helpful exploration where relevant into their socioeconomic status, other employment status, income (and especially poverty), sexual orientation, gender identity, discrimination and microaggressions, potentially traumatic events, violence and specifically intimate partner violence, depression, substance use, and negative interactions with the criminal justice system among others (Antebi-Gruszka et al., 2019) may be reasonable points of enquiry throughout the therapeutic relationship. Other factors like social isolation, community support, family, friends and professional networks are helpful enquiries when conducting ongoing assessment and a co-created care plan.

Where possible avoid taking a pathologising framework and instead consider a strengths-based exploration to discover what resources the sex worker–client already utilises and benefits from. Research overwhelmingly supports that therapy clients benefit when experiencing a sense of fair treatment and validation from their mental health care provider (Treloar et al., 2021). Research from sex workers has identified that some of the most effective forms of support experienced by sex workers to date have come not from mental health professionals but from their own communities and networks (Treloar et al., 2021). With this in mind, clinicians are encouraged to be especially attentive to workers who are experiencing isolation either personally and/or professionally, and consider encouraging them to make online sex worker connections if in-person options feel too risky.

Working with intersecting identities

As discussed previously, not all sex workers experience sex work the same way, nor do they experience stigma and discrimination the same way. This is especially relevant when we begin to unpack sex workers' multiple and intersecting identities, which may act as both sources of strength and power and/or further sources of shame and internalised self-criticism. For example, not all cis female sex workers are heterosexual nor identify as 'straight' despite their work exclusively servicing men. Simultaneously one's gender presentation while at work may be vastly different to one's gender presentation in other parts of their life. Similarly, one's other identities as parent, sibling, child, colleague, etc. may influence how someone sees themselves more than how they relate to their sex worker identity. Others again are adept at compartmentalising many parts of their lives in order to create a strong separation between work life and home life that may include practices like the following:

- Using a working name.
- Dressing differently at home and at work.
- Expressing one's gender differently.
- Using different speech, vocabulary or mannerisms.
- Using condoms at work but not at home with a partner.
- Enjoying alcohol and other substances at home recreationally but never at work or with clients.
- Engaging in particular sex acts with partners but never at work or vice versa.

Sometimes such compartmentalising can add to stress and stigma, especially if working incognito, while for others the distinctions are a form of self-care and professional boundary setting which should, in turn, be affirmed and encouraged. Clinicians may benefit from exploring the relationships between workers' intersecting identities as further sources of strength and resilience, especially where community and connection are sources of wellbeing.

Sex work, intimate partnerships and couple's counselling

Sex work stigma is pervasive in domestic, intimate partnerships too. As we have learned, the trouble with sex work is not the work itself, but how it uproots social order and flips power dynamics, making traditional models of relating less viable in these contexts.

There is very little research into the intimate partnerships of sex workers, and certainly none outside the context of relationship struggles, including harm, threats of harm and domestic violence (Johnson, 2019; Matos & Haze, 2019; Dickson, 2019). While such issues affect people in all kinds of relationships and sex workers in particular, it's important to recognise that sex workers' relationships can be tender, loving, fulfilling and powerful despite the social context the relationships exist in. Over the years of my work in counselling couples of many configurations, I have found that some of the struggles faced by sex workers and their partners in loving partnerships have been the result of typical relational complexities, not sex work itself. These topics include the following:

- Divisions of domestic labour (especially in heterosexual couples).
- The effects of patriarchy and gender expectations.
- Complex power dynamics.
- Needing support with boundaries.
- Emotional self-regulation and self-care.
- Communication skills including listening and patience.
- Developing empathy, tolerance and mindfulness.

However, what can make sex workers' intimate partnerships slightly more complicated than non–sex worker relationships is battling the stigma of their work *at home*. This can manifest when people struggle to accept their partners' sex working (especially when a sex worker is dating an allosexual or someone who experiences frequent sexual desire for their partner *and* jealousy when they are at work) and/or struggle to recognise the boundaries between 'work sex' with/for clients and 'at-home-sex' with a partner. From the clinician's perspective it can be easy to be tricked into thinking that if the sex working partner were to just quit and find a 'normal' job, the burden on the relationship would be lifted. It is not so straightforward. The issue is a relational dynamic with sex work as the presenting problem, but not the primary concern.

Relational issues that stem directly from one partner's sex work often speak to other issues within the relationship that benefit from both sex work stigma education and interventions drawn from the work of navigating consensual non-monogamies. While polyamory specialists are adept at working with relational complexities that usually centre love and multiple intimate ongoing relationships at their core, the wider spectrum of non-monogamies cover everything from casual hook-ups, swinging, 3, 4, 5somes, orgies to consensual multiple separate dating and beyond. The emphasis within couples therapy for sex workers and their jealous partners struggling with this dynamic may be more sex-focused and less intimacy/relationally focused.

For example, if couples are struggling with jealousy about the sex worker's sexual activities on the job, it may be helpful to initiate a conversation in couples counselling about how they define *love* in contrast with *sex*, and what both *love* and *sex* mean to the partnership in a loving relationship. For example:

- Is sex the only way you feel loved or express love?
- What does your partner do that makes you feel loved?
- What do you do to show your partner you love them?
- Where did you learn about love?
- Where did you learn about sex?
- When/How did you learn that they can coexist?
- When did you learn that they *must* coexist?
- Have you only ever experienced sex in the context of love?
- Have you ever experienced love and security without sex?
- What other areas of your life make you feel jealous?
- How do you manage those?

and so on.

Sometimes when clients are able to parse out the ways love and sex are different, they can explore strengthening the relationship by prioritising and privileging the areas of the relationship that make them feel confident (e.g. this is when I feel most loved by my partner) in contrast with the areas that make them feel insecure.

It can be helpful if the non–sex working partner is experiencing jealousy to have the opportunity to talk through their greatest fear – their worst-case scenarios. For example:

"I am afraid you're going to leave me"
"I am afraid you're going to get hurt at work"
"I am afraid you're having better sex at work than with me"

Sometimes when the fears are given the light of day, simply having them heard and validated can reduce their intensity. Similarly, partners may benefit from clinicians' guidance and support around the effects of sex work stigma and encourage the couple to develop a united front against stigma, rather than against each other. When couples can find ways to bond and unionise their love for each other, it can allow the relationship to flourish, while they recognise the enemy is not the partner or the partner's work, but the stigma, shame and mono-normative relationship structures that cause them to fight and feel insecure.

Similarly, allowing the sex working partner to explain how they feel about their work, about their partner's insecurities and what their ideal resolution might look like, allows the partners to find areas of shared bonding – both in joy and pain. For example, it's not uncommon for cohabiting couples where one is sex working to discover that they both feel anxious/uneasy when the sex working partner returns home from work. Or they both feel afraid that the relationship cannot sustain them. Or that they are both really proud of their partner's sex work and sex work activism and are both committed to battling stigma at home and on the streets, because their activism matters and bonds them together. When clinicians can help clients find ways that partners share burdens together, both painful and joyful, it can help lighten the load and reorient the fighting from personal attacks to political social justice strategy.

Fostering community care for better health outcomes

Overwhelmingly, research has highlighted that sex workers benefit the most from decriminalisation first and foremost and secondly finding support through their own peer networks and activist communities (Treloar et al., 2021). Such practices reduce the risk of harm imposed by isolation and encourage sex workers to seek support from each other, especially when working in isolated, regional or rural contexts (Scarlet Alliance, 1999; Treloar et al., 2021; Bloomquist & Sprankle, 2019). Such peer networks also offer location-specific, language-specific and culture-specific literature, health information, private listings of dangerous or suspect clients, mental and emotional health support plus camaraderie without shame. For sex workers who are historically mistrusting of traditional psychotherapy or who are afraid of being pathologised and misunderstood, peer support groups and events offer a wonderful opportunity for workers (and sometimes their partners) to discuss, explore and consider how they can ease the burden of stigma by sharing a laugh, a drink and resources while supporting themselves and their activism.

Conclusion

Sex workers are a unique sexual minority that share many common threads with the broader LGBTIQA+ and GSRD world. While being a stigmatised and marginalised group, they are a powerful and organised political force. Clinicians working with this community are best placed to draw on the same affirming clinical skills used with other sexual minorities while remaining sensitive to the unique legal position many sex workers find themselves in, with regard to personal freedom, safety, family, finances and other forms of social and professional discrimination.

Decriminalisation can reduce the impact on mental health to that of the general population, however the impact of stigma remains, and this is above all else what makes sex work a humanitarian issue, feminist issue, a social justice issue and a labour rights issue. As clinicians, it is our job to get educated, offer support and increase awareness by voicing our support for all sexual minorities while not overstepping the mark into interfering in sex workers' lives. When it comes to the work of sex work, like so many other areas of discrimination, the personal is political, and more than ever our support in terms of policy, advocacy and recognition of sovereignty matters.

References

Antebi-Gruszka, N., Spence, D., & Jendr, S. (2019). Guidelines for mental health practice with clients who engage in sex work. *Sexual and Relationship Therapy*, *34*(3), 339–354.

Benoit, C., Jansson, S. M., Smith, M., & Flagg, J. (2018). Prostitution stigma and its effect on the working conditions, personal lives, and health of sex workers. *Journal of Sex Research*, *55*(4–5), 457–471.

Benoit, C., McCarthy, B., & Jansson, M. (2015). Occupational stigma and mental health: Discrimination and depressions among front-line service workers. *Canadian Public Policy*, *41*(Supplement 2), S61–S69.

Bloomquist, K., & Sprankle, E. (2019). Sex worker affirmative therapy: Conceptualization and case study. *Journal of Sexual and Relationship Therapy*, *34*(3), 392–408.

CDC, Center for Disease Control. (2019). *HIV Risk Among Persons Who Exchange Sex for Money or Nonmonetary Items* [Online]. Retrieved November 6, 2021, from www.cdc.gov/hiv/group/sexworkers.html

Center for Health and Gender Equity. (2016). *U.S. Foreign Assistance and SRHR of Female Sex Workers*. s.l. Retrieved from https://srhrforall.org/all-women-all-rights-sex-workers-includedu-s-foreign-assistance-and-srhr-of-female-sex-workers/

Dickson, H. (2019). Sex work, motherhood and stigma. *Sex and Relationship Therapy*, *34*(3), 332–334.

Donovan, B., et al. (2012). *The Sex Industry in New South Wales: A Report to the NSW Ministry of Health*. Sydney: Kirby Institute. University of New South Wales.

Dworkin, A. (1981). *Pornography: Men Possessing Women*. New York: Plume.

Farley, M., & Barkan, H. (1998). Prostitution, violence, and posttraumatic stress disorder. *Women Health*, *27*(3), 37–49.

Geymonat, G. G., Macioti, P. G., & Mai, N. (2021). *Sex Work and Mental Health; Access to Mental Health Services for People Who Sell Sex in Germany, Italy, Sweden, and UK*. Berlin: Public Health Fund of the Open Society Foundations.

Goffman, E. (1963). *Stigma: Notes on the Management of Spoilt Identity*. Englewood Cliffs, NJ: Prentice-Hall Inc.

Goldenberg, S. M., Thomas, R. M., Forbes, A., & Baral, S. (2021). *Sex Work, Health and Human Rights. Global Inequities, Challenges, and Opportunities for Action*. s.l.: Springer.

Grant, M. G. (2014). *Playing the Whore: The Work of Sex Work*. London: Verso.

Harcourt, C., et al. (2010). The decriminalisation of prostitution is associated with better coverage of health promotion programs for sex workers. *Australian & New Zealand Journal of Public Health*, *34*(5), 482–486.

Hatzenbuehler, M. L. (2009). How does sexual minority stigma "get under the skin?" A psychological mediation framework. *Psychological Bulletin*, *135*, 707–730.

Jeffreys, E. (2009). NSWP: Sex worker-driven research: best practice ethics. *Challenging Politics Critical Voices* [Online]. Retrieved November 5, 2021, from www.nswp.org/sites/nswp.org/files/Elena-Jeffreys-Sex-Worker-Driven-Research-1.pdf

Johnson, J. (2019). Dating while sex working: Civilian dates carry more risk for sex workers. *Sexual and Relationship Therapy*, *34*(3), 329–331.

Koken, J. (2012). Independent female escort's strategies for coping with sex work-related stigma. *Sexuality & Culture*, *16*(3), 209–229.

Langdridge, D. (2007). Gay affirmative therapy: A theoretical framework and defense. *Journal of Gay and Lesbian Psychotherapy*, *11*(1–2), 27–43.

Matos, B., & Haze, L. (2019). Bottoms up: A whorelistic literature review and commentary on sex workers' romantic relationships. *Sexual and Relationship Therapy*, *34*(3), 372–391.

Pedersen, A. C., Stenersen, M. R., & Bridges, S. K. (2019). Toward affirming therapy: What sex workers want and need from mental health providers. *Journal of Positive Psychology*, 1–20.

Rayson, J., & Alba, B. (2019). Experiences of stigma and discrimination as predictors of mental health help-seeking among sex workers. *Sexual and Relationship Therapy*, *34*(3), 277–289.

Rhodes, T., et al. (2008). Police violence and sexual risk among female and transvestite sex workers in Serbia. *BMJ*, *337*.

Rule, R., & Twinley, R. (2021). Developing an occupational perspective of women involved in sex work: A discussion paper. *Journal of Occupational Science*, *28*(1), 133–143.

Sawicki, D. A., Meffert, B. N., Read, K., & Heinz, A. J. (2019). Culturally competent health care for sex workers: An examination of myths that stigmatize sex work and hinder access to care. *Sex and Relationship Therapy*, *34*(3), 355–371.

Scarlet Alliance. (1999). *Unjust and Counter-Productive: The Failure of Government to Protect Sex Workers from Discrimination*. s.l. Retrieved from ww.scarletalliance.org.au

Seib, C., Fischer, J., & Najman, J. (2009). The health of female sex workers from three industry sectors in Queensland, Australia. *Social Science and Medicine*, *68*(3), 473–478.

Shannon, K., & Csete, J. (2010). Violence, condom negotiation, and HIV/STI risk among sex workers. *JAMA*, *304*(5), 573–574.

Treloar, C., Stardust, Z., Cama, E., & Kim, J. (2021). Rethinking the relationship between sex work, mental health and stigma: A qualitative Study of Sex Workers in Australia. *Social Science and Medicine*, *268*.

U.S Department of State. (2004). *Trafficking in Persons Report*. s.l. Retrieved from www.hsdl.org/?view&did=454934

van Anders, S. M. (2015). Beyond sexual orientation: Integrating gender/sex and diverse sexualities via sexual configurations theory. *Archives of Sexual Behavior*, *44*, 1177–1213.

Vanwesenbeek, I. (2001). Another decade of social scientific work on sex work: A review of research 1990–2000. *Annual Review of Sex Research*, *12*, 242–289.

Appendix I

- Agustın, L. M. (2007). Sex at the margins: Migration, labour markets, and the rescue industry. London: Zed Books.
- Chateauvert, M. (2014). Sex workers unite: A history of the movement from Stonewall to SlutWalk. Boston, MA: Beacon Press.
- Davina, L. (2017). Thriving in sex work: Heartfelt advice for staying sane in the sex industry. Oakland, CA: The Erotic as Power Press.
- Grant, M.G. (2014). Playing The Whore: The Work of Sex Work. London. Verso.
- Lee, J. (2015). Coming out like a porn star: Essays on pornography, protection, and privacy. Los Angeles, CA: Three L Media.

Chapter 5

The trans compass

A way of hearing and understanding trans people's relationships with their identities

Ellis Morgan

Trans affirmative therapy with clients considering or undertaking a gender transition often involves supportive exploration of what it might mean for them to live with a greater sense of gender congruence. In this chapter, I suggest that affirmative work of this kind is greatly benefitted by an informed perspective toward the struggle for gender legitimacy that trans people universally face and an ability to hear the varied ways that these struggles can interplay with their ways of being understood by themselves and others. I offer a therapeutic tool called the Trans Compass. The tool provides a simple, effective way of readily locating some essential features of trans clients' shifting relationships with their gender and their transness as they consider and move through gender transition. Beyond this, however, it can also help us understand how gender legitimacy struggles can profoundly affect every aspect of our trans clients' emotional, practical and relational worlds.

The Trans Compass tool enters the therapeutic field when vociferous public and professional debates continue about the nature of sex and gender, the validity of transness and the role of therapists in facilitating or 'challenging' clients who seek gender transition (see Morgan & Nicholson, 2023). This chapter does not seek to add to these debates. Instead, it takes for granted the right of all people to determine the gender that feels most fitting and congruent for them at any given time in their lives. For therapists using the Trans Compass, this initial leap from scepticism to trust in our clients' right to self-define their gender must be taken before any of its further orientating potentials can be used.

The foundations of the trans compass – trans legitimacy stress and the drive toward gender congruence

In December 2014, international news broke that an American transgender seventeen-year-old, Leelah Alcorn, had taken her own life, publishing a poignant suicide note on social media just before her death (Jennings, 2015). Leelah had been seeking support for a gender transition, but disastrously, she was sent to a Christian conversion camp instead, culminating in her death. The insidious effects

DOI: 10.4324/9781003260561-6

of the anti-trans messaging were clear within the note she left; 'I'm never going to transition successfully', she wrote. 'Either I live the rest of my life as a lonely man who wishes he were a woman or I live my life as a lonelier woman who hates herself. There's no winning. There's no way out'. Leelah felt agonisingly caught between her desire to live with a sense of gender congruence as a woman, and the internalised message that such a life could never truly be a 'success'.

In their most extreme and painful form, Leelah's feelings exemplify what I have come to see as two defining features of transgender experience. One is the desire to redefine one's birth-assigned gender to live with a greater sense of gender congruence. The other is encountering the uncomfortable social friction that always accompanies, to some degree, trans people's efforts towards this. I have come to think of this second feature of transgender experience as giving rise to a distinct, recognisable phenomenon that might aptly be called *gender legitimacy stress*; the psychological impact of living in a social context where your gender is pervasively regarded as being less 'real' than those of cisgender people.

Gender legitimacy stress can take many guises. For many, living with an uncertain or fragile sense of one's social gender validity affects feelings of belonging, self-value and safety. For others, there may be difficulty in accepting the legitimacy of one's own gender. Sometimes it takes the form of occasional background worries, at other times it takes the form of overt and frequent social panic. Often, it manifests as the emotional accompaniment to everyday legitimacy stressors: someone holding their pee for hours for fear of using a public toilet; a person worrying about when to disclose that they are trans on a date; a non-binary person experiencing frequent misgendering in at least some of their personal relationships or in public spaces.

Legitimacy stress can be considered a variant of 'minority stress' (Meyer, 2003), but the two concepts are not interchangeable. Minority stress is a much broader category, encompassing the many ways that structural disadvantage presses on the lives of minority groups. By separating the concept of legitimacy stress from minority stress, I am suggesting that there are different ways that structural disadvantage can operate; as social demotion (where you are seen as *unequal* to a majority or privileged group) and as social illegitimacy (where you are seen as less *entitled to your identity* than a majority or privileged group). Some forms of social marginalisation involve experiencing one of these, and some involve experiencing both. Thought of in this way, it is possible to see that many other varieties of legitimacy stress also circulate in society; for example, a Black British person who is often asked 'but where are you really from?' or an adoptive parent who is used to being told that she is not a 'real' mum. As a society, we have a habit of thinking that there are specific paths to being 'real' in many areas of life. It is important for therapists working with transgender clients to recognise the powerful and persistent way this occurs in relation to gender identity.

To begin to look more closely at what this means for our therapeutic work with trans clients, we need to engage with two fundamental aspects of gender transition that work to create the Trans Compass.

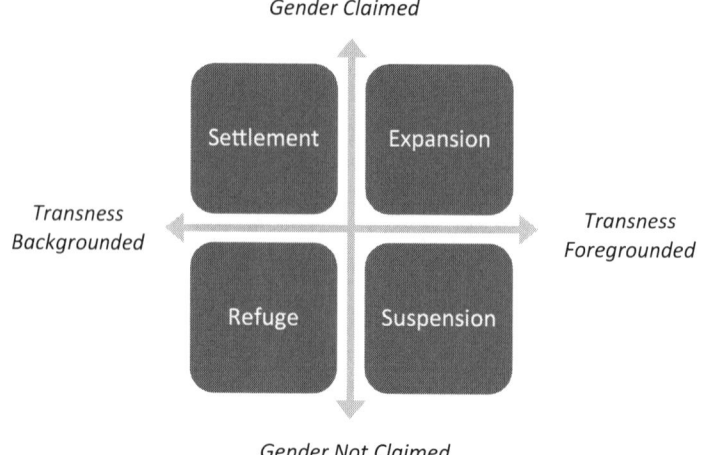

Figure 5.1 The trans compass.

Self-claiming gender: the north and south of the trans compass

The first defining feature of the Trans Compass is a recognition that coming to live with a greater sense of gender congruence involves making a *personal claim* to a new gender identity. Often, the beginning stages of transition are focused on exploring which gender might feel more fitting for us than the one we were assigned at birth. But just beyond this, there is the often fraught matter of coming to feel personally entitled to make a claim to that new gender identity. It is the critical gear change from saying something like 'identifying as a woman would be more fitting for me' to saying 'I am a woman'. It is a profound and often challenging shift, given the legitimacy issues that are endemic to trans identities.

My work with trans clients over the years has shown me that there are no certainties about how this process of personal identity claiming will play out in any given context. Sometimes people's claiming of their new gender identity is confident and speedy, and at other times it is a struggle so great that it never gets off the ground at all. Despite this variability, when processes of transition are being discussed in any domain – be it therapeutic, medical, academic or cultural – it seems that this important stage is often glossed over. Instead, it is imagined that transition processes involve an initial exploration and decision-making process (i.e. whether to go ahead with transition) followed by a purely social process of identity negotiation. In my practice I see many people going ahead with a decision to undertake some form of medical or social transition despite their continued struggle to self-claim their own gender identity. And I also see many people not taking steps toward medical or social transition, despite wanting to do so, because of the seeming impossibility of ever feeling valid within the gender they feel would be most fitting for them.

The Trans Compass tool centralises this important variability within trans people's feelings of entitlement to claim their congruent gender. It is represented by a vertical axis, showing a continuum of feelings toward 'claiming' or 'not claiming' one's gender – whether this is one that is binary or non-binary or a confident claiming of being non-gendered. In reality, of course, claiming gender is rarely a clear-cut matter for trans people; we can have mixed feelings about it and feel entitled to our identities in some moments, and not in others. However, for the sake of simplicity, the 'claiming gender' axis delineates a rough generalisation of our feelings toward gender legitimacy, which can then enable deeper discussion about the complexities that we can experience within this.

Positioning transness: the east and west of the trans compass

The second defining feature of the Trans Compass is a recognition that from the point that a person acknowledges to themselves that there is a discrepancy between their birth-assigned gender and their congruent gender, being trans becomes a potentially relevant part of their identity. Here, I am using the term 'trans' in the most inclusive sense. It is sometimes the case that non-binary people find that the terminology of transness is too heavy with the implication of a binary transition to be fitting for them (see, for example, Darwin, 2020) – but in the sense that I mean it here, 'transness' can also be read as an arising sense of queer gender difference from cisgender people.

A great deal of social research has documented the many different perspectives that trans people can have toward their trans identity and the sense of difference from cisgender people it can create (e.g. Hines & Sanger, 2010). Whilst for some people transness is regarded as a merely incidental biographical fact, for others, it can become a central aspect of their sense of self, and it can have important implications for how a person seeks to be understood. On the Trans Compass, how 'backgrounded' or 'foregrounded' transness is within a person's identity is represented on a horizontal axis – and again is a simplification of what, in reality, can often be complex and mixed feelings, for the sake of creating a discursive tool. Together, the two axes form a quadrant diagram, identifying what we might loosely think of as four generalised and changeable trans identity situations. It is important to be clear that these 'situations' do not define four specific trans identities, but rather four broadly recognisable ways that, as trans people, we might *relate* to our gender and transness at any point in time. On the Trans Compass, each of these identity situations is named to represent something of its character.

Gender settlement: claiming gender, backgrounding trans difference

For many of the clients I see, a way of relating to gender and transness as a form of *settlement* is obvious from the outset. It is the kind of perspective we hear when someone articulates both a sense of entitlement to their congruent gender, and a desire for that gender to be understood in the same uncomplicated way that a cisgender person would likely have their gender understood. In the language of the Trans Compass, their transness is only of 'backgrounded' relevance to the way they understand their gender. One of my clients summed it up well when he said to me 'my maleness is just the same as any other man's maleness. I just had to transition to get here'. It does not mean that a person necessarily rejects transness as an identity, but more that they don't want it to interfere with how their gender is made sense of and understood.

Whilst the desire for gendered settlement might sound straightforward and probably familiar as a trans perspective, there is a great deal of legitimacy stress that can sometimes surface in attempting to make it a personal reality. My client Alison learned this only too well as part of her gender transition. I remember her saying 'I know this won't be easy, because I'll never pass, but I can't live my life without doing this'. She described her fantasy that one day she could tell a new person in her life that she is trans and for them to say 'Oh I had no idea' – and then for them to continue to treat her just the way they had before. It is important to appreciate that not all trans people want to socially 'pass' as cisgender and that 'passing' by no means guarantees that any trans person will be seen as legitimate, by themselves or those around them. But especially when gender settlement is desired, it can be of huge significance to trans people's lives. On the surface, Alison was stoical about the fact she felt this would always remain a dream, but the legitimacy stress it left her with was palpable in how she would attempt to compensate for it in other ways. She described how she would anxiously monitor her way of dressing in a way that was feminine, but conservative enough not to cause a stir. She would hold herself back from talking too often in work meetings or social situations, for fear of appearing too confident, which she feared could be perceived as masculine. She would avoid women-only spaces, including public toilets to circumvent the painful situation of having to publicly protest her legitimacy. Alison's deepest desire was to get on with her life as a woman, just like any other, but she felt she had to continually fight against being seen as an interloper; someone who would always be marked as different. Alison's daily experiences as a visible trans woman fed her perspective that her transness would never be the 'backgrounded' part of her identity that she desired for it to be.

For those people who desire the sense of gender ordinariness that defines gender settlement, but whose transness is less visibly noticeable, the legitimacy issues they face can take a very different form. My client Craig was in such a situation when he approached me for therapy. He had transitioned many years before and had moved to a new city to escape the small village where he grew up and had transitioned, and where he had felt hyper-visible as a trans person. Craig craved the sense of gender ordinariness that living without his transness being known would afford him, but as he was to discover, it left him with a crippling sense of isolation. Gender transition had been an important part of his life experience, even if it didn't change the way he wanted his maleness understood. Craig was left with what I have come to see as a common gender settlement legitimacy dilemma; if he didn't come out to his new friends, Craig felt he would never feel fully known in terms of his life experience or realise the deeper potential of his friendships. But, if he were to come out as trans, it would mean taking the huge risk that those friends may no longer grant him the unproblematic legitimacy as a man that he currently experienced.

Whilst a desire to be understood through a lens of gender settlement is more common for binary trans people, it can also be desired by some people with less binary identities. Here the challenge is obvious; achieving a sense of taken-for-granted gender belonging is difficult when your gender itself is seen by society as an anomaly. My client Kris felt in such a position. For Kris, like many people, neither a male nor female identity felt comfortable or authentic. The difficulty for Kris, however, was that they were resistant to inhabiting a non-binary gender because they didn't want the sense of 'otherness' that they felt would inevitably accompany such a socially contentious gender identity. 'The truth is, I'm non-binary, but I just want for people to recognise that my gender is no more radical than anyone else's' Kris would tell me. Their anguish was understandable; taking on the mantel of overt transness or queer difference can feel like a burden for those who desire the ordinariness of gendered settlement.

Kris's solution was to socially transition to a non-binary gender but deliberately lean toward a distinctively female or male self-presentation when they felt they needed a safer social identity to retreat to. This solution came with its challenges; the legitimacy stress of constantly adapting their presentation to conform to gendered norms was not so different from Alison's stress of keeping her language and dress in check to try to be accepted as a woman, or Craig's careful selection of who he should and shouldn't come out to, to retain his sense of social legitimacy as a man. The thread that runs through all of them is the core gender settlement dilemma that we must be sensitive to as therapists; wanting to feel known, and wanting to belong uncomplicatedly, and yet feeling the often impossible tension between the two.

Gender expansion: claiming gender, foregrounding trans difference

As trans people have become increasingly visible over the last two decades, we have seen a great proliferation in the kinds of gender identities that people feel able to claim for themselves (e.g. Munro, 2019). For many of these more nuanced ways of defining one's gendered reality, a key theme is embracing the queer difference that comes with a gender that has been redefined. In terms of the Trans Compass, this embracing of difference alongside a claiming of one's gender is understood as expressing a desire to be seen through a lens of gender expansion. For some trans people this desire to be understood in an expansive way can be subtle, where they see their trans history or experience as being a valued, contouring facet of a gender that is otherwise similar to those of cisgender people. For others it is a more radically queer, deliberately differentiated gender.

When Jez emailed me about starting therapy, and described himself as a genderqueer trans man, I was conscious that I would need to hear more to understand quite what this meant to him. He arrived for his first session in a smart shirt and corduroy trousers and had a quiet, unassuming manner. Outwardly at least, Jez had a fairly conventional male appearance, and to understand what his genderqueerness meant to him, it was clear that one needed to dig deeper than visuals alone.

'It took a while to work out my own way of being trans' Jez described to me.

> At first, I just wanted to be a man. But as I transitioned and started feeling more comfortable in my own skin, the more I felt able to relax and just be me. Although I like to be perceived as male in public, I'm more comfortable when people closer to me know that I'm not just male. It's only really when people see all the mixed ways that being trans effects who I am, that I feel that they see me.

As Jez talked, it became clear to me that he sees his gender through a lens of gender expansion. Whilst he at least partially identifies with maleness, he also feels queerly trans-different from that. For him the very meaning of his maleness was contoured by his transness. The legitimacy issues that arose for him centred on his fear that the security that an uncomplicatedly male identity afforded him would be disrupted if he disclosed his more complex gender identity to others. Jez held an ambition to become a priest – but he was extremely concerned that his genderqueerness might be controversial in the eyes of his church. 'I'm already out as a trans man in the church', he told me, 'and everyone is fine with it, but if I really explained about how I feel about my gender, there would definitely be people who would want to veto that, in terms of how it looks to the public'.

Jez, like Craig, eventually found his way forward by being more open with some people within his church than others. But we can see that the nature of the gender expansion dilemma is distinct from the gender settlement dilemma; whilst for Craig, the difficulty was around telling people that he was trans, for Jez the difficulty was telling people about *the significance* of his being trans, and specifically how it shaped the meaning of his gender.

In Jez's case, the fact he described himself as a genderqueer trans man was a clue that he wanted for his gender to be understood in an expansive way, but we can't always rely on these kinds of prompts. Often, I will work with clients whose way of talking about their gender would initially suggest a gender settlement way of wanting to be understood. However, on listening more deeply to them, it becomes clear that this assumption would miss important aspects of their feelings that point towards a more differentiated, trans-contoured way of wanting for their gender to be understood. The important thing to remember is that the gendered associations we have for any trans client's name, pronoun or gender label is never enough on its own to tell us how they want their gender – and its relationship with their transness – to be understood. There is *always* deeper listening required to give us this steer.

Whilst a desire for gender settlement carries the difficulty of being granted legitimacy within the conventional 'mould' of femaleness or maleness, gender expansion has the further complication of being granted legitimacy when you try to bend that mould into a new shape – or reject it altogether. For those people with non-binary genders that depart more radically from identifications of maleness or femaleness, legitimacy issues take on a different character still. Where those seeking to be understood as some variety of female or male often have to argue for their entitlement to their gendered belonging, non-binary people are in the unenviable position of having to argue for the very *existence* of their gender. The legitimacy issues faced by non-binary people are evident within the fundamental structures of our society; everyday language, including pronouns, essential public spaces such as toilets, and official documentation such as passports are all divided by binary gender norms. But beyond this, non-binary people find themselves freshly negotiating their gendered meaning in each new relationship they form, with no ready template to make their genders legible. Like Jez, who often decided to present himself as more conventionally male than his gender identity was, many non-binary people pick and choose when it feels 'worth it' to enter these daily battles for legitimacy and recognition. After all, being understood expansively is only possible when we encounter those willing to see in an expansive way.

Gender suspension: not claiming gender, foregrounding trans difference

The perspectives of gender settlement and gender expansion outlined so far both encompass the legitimacy issues that trans people encounter when trans people's congruent, claimed genders are not fully understood or taken seriously by others. Within gender suspension (and in the following section, 'gender refuge'), there is a departure from this, and instead, we encounter the perspectives of trans people for whom legitimacy issues mean that even claiming their congruent gender themselves can feel too difficult. When this difficulty intersects with a desire (or perhaps a pragmatic willingness) to foreground a trans identity instead, we are in the territory of gender suspension.

My client Billy was someone for whom the relationship with their gender and transness would best be described as gender suspension. Billy came to see me to explore her desires to transition from male to female, and over the course of her therapy we worked through the complexities of her desires, fears and hopes that surrounded this. But as she made the decision to progress with a medical and social transition, it was clear that Billy – like many of my clients – struggled to feel entitled to self-claim her new gender. 'I just don't feel I can sit here and say I'm a woman', I would hear her say. 'I'm definitely not a man, and maybe one day, when I'm further down the line, I'll be able to hold my head high and say I'm a woman now, but for now I think all I can really say is that I'm trans'.

When clients struggle in this way I can absolutely understand the nature of their difficulty. It is extremely challenging not to internalise the social messaging that being trans, at best, creates a pathway to a substandard version of your gender, or at worst, creates a mirage of a gender that can never be considered genuine. In my work I often find there is an important conversation to be had when clients are experiencing this struggle, to uncover the specific variety of legitimacy stress at play. What in their mind, I wonder, would it take to be able to make a personal claim to their congruent gender? Some might feel that they need to have taken enough tangible medical or social steps to feel they've 'earned it'. Others might feel they need to look in the mirror and see what they believe looks 'enough' like a newly gendered version of themselves. Others still might feel that at least some other people in their lives unproblematically read them as their new gender. Though, for some, the difficult truth is that they suspect that their gnawing sense of being a gender-outsider might never allow them a sense of true belonging.

Whilst in an ideal world all trans people would feel a sense of entitlement to claim whatever gender identity feels congruent for them at any given time, in my practice I often perceive that a client's willingness to embrace their trans-ness as a kind of placeholder whilst they work towards a sense of gender entitle-ment can, at least, be a silver lining in these situations. My client Billy felt 'shored up' by her trans identity; it allowed her to let go of her misfitting male gender identity without completely letting go of any kind of gendered belong-ing. Alongside this, I often see how especially when a new gender identity feels precarious, embracing a trans identity can provide a crucial sense of both com-munity and personhood.

For any trans person who is clear about the gender identity that feels desirable and congruent for them but struggles to feel 'enough' to claim it, the legitimacy stress they face is clear; a deep internalised sense of gender displacement. There can be some respite from these difficult feelings for those who embrace a trans identity despite this absence of a claimed gender identity. However, as we will see in the next section, for those who don't, the situation can be far more challenging.

Gender refuge: not claiming gender, backgrounding trans difference

So far, I have set out the kinds of relationships that people form with their gender and transness, when at least one of these is claimed, or brought further to the foreground within their identity. In this final quadrant we encounter the kinds of situations that arise when legitimacy struggles mean that people feel unable to claim a new gender, but where they also feel that it is too unsafe or too undesirable to foreground transness as an aspect of their identity. This is the uncomfortable position of gender refuge.

In these situations, given that transness does not offer someone the 'holding place' that we see within gender suspension, instead people often find themselves without any way of comfortably relating to and identifying their gendered selves. In my experience, such an absence can be extremely unsettling and disorientating for people, and understandably, the natural response is for alternative 'refuges' to be sought out; and unfortunately, the 'refuges' found are often equally undesirable and all too often unsafe harbours.

Earlier in this chapter I talked about Leelah Alcorn, who took her own life after becoming convinced that she could never live the life that she so deeply desired within her congruent gender. For her the ultimate 'refuge' from her situation was death. The high suicide rates amongst trans populations are testament to the fact that Leelah is far from alone in seeking this ultimate escape from feeling one's congruent gender will always remain impossibly out of reach (e.g. McNeil et al., 2012; Testa et al., 2017). Of course, it will certainly be the case that many trans people who have taken their lives have felt able to claim their genders at least some of the time, and others will have felt a sense of proud affiliation with a trans identity. But it is also very likely that many will have taken their lives because of this seemingly insurmountable feeling that the identity they most craved for themselves felt like an impossibility, and for whom death became a preferable option.

Fortunately, in my experience, there are other refuges that people find for themselves besides suicide, though all of them involve a painful degree of compromise. Sometimes a person may decide that transition is too risky, and remain living as their birth assigned gender, some or all of the time. In other cases, a person might compromise and transition to a gender that feels safer or more achievable, though not the one that truly feels congruent for them. Sometimes, like for my client Rowan, all of these are tried at different times, as they try out one compromise after another, trying to find a way of living that feels least painful.

Rowan was assigned male at birth and transitioned for the first time in her early twenties, responding to her deeply held longing to live within her congruent gender as female. This first transition brought Rowan a degree of comfort and fulfilment for a short time, and in our sessions she looked back on that time with a nostalgic glow. However, the comfort had been short lived, as Rowan found herself crippled with feelings of anxiety and illegitimacy fed by ridicule and transphobic abuse that she routinely faced in her life; local residents in her area who had known Rowan throughout her transition intimidated her whenever she left her house and began putting everything from dog faeces to lit fireworks through her letterbox. Rowan was rehomed by the council to escape the abuse, but the fear and internalised sense of illegitimacy stayed with her. Within five years Rowan made the painful decision to transition back to male. As she put it 'no-one, including me will ever take me seriously as a woman, so I may as well face my reality that I'm left with living as a man'.

Since this time Rowan had attempted living as a woman once again for a period of six months, but again she encountered debilitating feelings of fear, shame and lack and retreated to the uncomfortable 'refuge' of maleness. This was the point at which we began our sessions together and started to work through this painful experience and address the difficult matter of how Rowan might find a way of living more comfortably. As Rowan unpacked her experience, it became clear that a life lived in the thick of transphobia had made it difficult for her to ever spend time looking at her relationship with herself, and her gender as part of this. The only way through it was to begin to tease apart the feelings she had about her own sense of gender, from the incessant social messaging she received about the gender that felt permissible for her.

Both Leelah Alcorn and my client Rowan faced stark choices in their search for a refuge in the context of feeling adrift from their congruent gender. For many others who I work with, there are more subtle ways that a search for a refuge can play out, as they seek identities that feel more possible or accessible than the congruent gender that they would otherwise claim for themselves. For example, I often work with clients who would ideally identify their redefined gender in a binary male or female way but, given their struggle to feel that they will ever truly 'make the grade', come to claim socially – or take 'refuge' in – a non-binary gender instead, feeling some relief from the lack of social template it comes with. Conversely, I work with many people who feel that the gender that would be most accurate and fitting for them would be non-binary, but claim – or take 'refuge' in – a binary gender instead, because of their struggle to imagine this as a realistic possibility for themselves. As one of my clients put it 'where I'm from, you just can't live like that'.

Whatever 'refuge' is being sought when our clients find themselves in these situations, our role as therapists can be vital: in providing a companion as options are considered, hope in the possibility that a liveable, self-legitimised life can be found, and amongst all of this, the certain sense that at least one other person can understand, and find to be legitimate, the gendered belonging that seems so elusive in the rest of their life.

Therapy beyond borders

In offering the Trans Compass as a therapeutic tool, my hope is that as therapists, we can more readily offer recognition and empathic understanding to our trans clients of the kinds of legitimacy struggles that they face, and the ways that their situations and identities become shaped by these struggles. All too often, it is easy to imagine that trans people unproblematically step into and freely communicate the gender identities that they most desire and feel most fitting for them; but this misses the huge task that trans people can face in fighting against the tide of socially-contested belonging. Who gets to fit particular gender categories, in what instances, remains a matter of ongoing politicised public debate, and one that plays out in trans people's everyday lives. Unsurprisingly these debates are frequently internalised by trans people themselves, leading to difficulties in claiming their genders, and complexities in navigating their relationships and the social spaces they find themselves in.

My hope too is that as therapeutic practitioners we remain aware of the ways in which transness, as an identity in its own right, can be held in different ways by different people who come to redefine their gender. For some, there is a great desire for transness to be held lightly in terms of its influence on their gendered meaning. For others, it is a critical, contouring facet of how they want their genders to be understood. For others still, it becomes a vital way of being recognised, when legitimacy issues mean that laying claim to a new gender feels too far out of reach. And finally, my wish is that as a profession and as a society we might begin to notice an entire section of the trans community who are often erased through a lack of attention to trans legitimacy issues; those who never quite feel able to move into their congruent genders, but seek a quiet and often uncomfortable refuge between identities and communities.

Putting the knowledge contained in the Trans Compass into practice is, in reality, a subtle and nuanced matter in our therapeutic work. Our trans clients are often likely to have complex feelings about their gender and transness, and no one fits neatly into one of these relational categories in a static way, all the time. Like all feelings, a trans person's sense of gender legitimacy or trans identity will shift over time and from one context to another; people often make 'sort of' claims to gender and have conflicting feelings about whether their transness is essential to who they are. Rather than erase this complexity, the tool is intended to provide a starting point for more discussion around the intricacies of our relationships with our identities.

From my therapeutic perspective, it is not important that we accurately 'diagnose' which of the four quadrants our client's relationship with their gender and transness points to, but rather that we bear it in mind as a steer towards hearing more astutely the ways that clients might feel about themselves and want to be understood. Rather than 'fixing' clients in place as talking from one perspective or another, that might mean continually moving with them as they reveal all the contrasting ways they can feel about themselves. I know that as a trans person myself, there have been times in my own life when my transness has felt central to the way that I want my gender understood. And there have been other times, and other relational situations, where my transness has very much faded into the background – and even times when the gender that I want to be recognised as has shifted in its meaning. Perhaps the most challenging thing we face then in engaging in this work is being able to legitimise our gender diverse clients in whatever way they are relating to themselves at any given point in time, without holding onto one version of their gender or transness as being the one that 'really' defines them. It is only with this kind of flexible recognition and legitimisation that we can truly be with, and value, our clients in all their complexity.

References

Darwin, H. (2020). Challenging the cisgender/transgender binary: Nonbinary people and the transgender label. *Gender and Society*, *34*(3), 357–380.

Hines, S., & Sanger, T. (2010). *Transgender Identities: Towards a Social Analysis of Gender Identity*. New York: Routledge.

Jennings, K. (2015). Leelah Alcorn and the continued struggle for equity for LGBT students. *The Educational Forum*, *4*(79), 343–345.

McNeil, J., Bailey, L., Ellis, S., & Regan, M. (2012). *Trans Mental Health Study*. Retrieved from www.treverseresearch.com/wp-content/uploads/2012/12/Mental-Health-2012.pdf

Meyer, I. H. (2003). Prejudice, social stress and mental health in lesbian, gay and bisexual populations: Conceptual issues and research evidence. *Psychological Bulletin, 129*(5), 674–697.

Morgan, E., & Nicholson, S. (2023). Trans sex: A practitioners dialogue. In S. Neves & D. Davies (Eds.), *Erotically Queer*. Abingdon, OX: Routledge.

Munro, S. (2019). Non-binary and genderqueer: An overview of the field. *International Journal of Transgenderism, 20*(2–3), 126–131.

Testa, R. J., Michaels, M. S., Bliss, W., Rogers, M. L., Balsam, K. F., & Joiner, T. (2017). Suicidal ideation in transgender people: Gender minority stress and interpersonal theory factors. *Journal of Abnormal Psychology, 126*(1), 125–136.

Chapter 6

Working with bi+ clients
Considerations for individual and relationship therapy

Dr Susannah Grant

Overview of the chapter

This chapter focuses on working with clients who are, or have the potential to be, attracted to more than one gender. In discussing this lived experience, this chapter refers to terms cited by literature, or uses 'bi+' as an inclusive umbrella term. Whilst this chapter can't offer a one-size-fits-all guide to working with all clients who have bi+ lived experience, the intention is to increase awareness so that as a therapist, you can practise in a more informed, affirmative, and anti-oppressive way.

Introduction: bi+ identities and lived experience

Historically, the term 'bisexual' has been used to convey the lived experience of being attracted to more than one gender. Today, exactly how to define bisexuality, and other non-monosexual identities, continues to be discussed and unfold. In recent years, alongside the term *bisexual*, other identity labels have arisen: both as umbrella terms, and alternative labels which highlight specific aspects of this lived experience (Galupo, 2018). Inclusive umbrella labels you may come across are non-monosexual, plurisexual, bi+, queer, and multisexual-spectrum (mspec).

Specific labels you may come across are outlined in Table 6.1, however, the meanings ascribed to particular labels may well shift from client to client.

Table 6.1 Identity labels and possible meanings

Specific labels	Possible meaning: attraction...
Bisexual	To more than one gender; the same gender as myself and different genders
Pansexual	To all genders, regardless of gender
Sexually fluid	Shifts over time (in any time frame and in any way)
Polysexual	To many genders
Omnisexual	To all genders, not regardless of gender
Other terms: bi-curious, hetero-flexible, homo-flexible, lesbi-flexible and others	May convey curiosity, flexibility, or a learning towards one identity, for example

DOI: 10.4324/9781003260561-7

Clients may also bring their own definitions and labels, or describe an attraction to, or sexual behaviour with, individuals of more than one gender, but identify as gay, lesbian, or heterosexual; or proactively choose not to label themselves at all. They may also prefer to break down their romantic and sexual attraction more specifically (e.g. biromantic, demisexual).

Prevalence

Whilst past research generally conflated bisexual research with other orientations (GB, LB, LGB, for example), recent years have seen significant change. We now have a better understanding of both the lived experience and the difficulties faced by bi+ people.

Reports regarding the prevalence of bi+ people understandably differ across different measures. In the US, the 'Invisible Minority' report (2016) indicated that bisexual people make up 52% of the LGBT community. In the UK, YouGov's (2015) survey showed that 23% of people state they are not 100% heterosexual; rising to 49% for young people (Dahlgreen & Shakespeare, 2015). The Bisexuality Report (2012) indicated that in the US, 3–5% self-identify as bisexual, 13% of women and 6% of men state their attraction to more than one gender, and referred to Kinsey's research that found that many people were not exclusively behaviourally monosexual.

Different models and measures of sexual orientation provide alternative lenses with which to view bi+ experience (see Swan, 2018, for an in-depth examination), and clients in therapy may describe bi+ lived experience in many different ways. If this is viewed through the Klein Grid (1993), for example, aspects of the experience might include sexual attraction, sexual behaviour, sexual fantasies, emotional preference, social preference, lifestyle, and self-identification. Clients might describe shifts in one or many of these aspects over time, which aligns with Klein, as well as later literature regarding sexual fluidity over time and spaces (Diamond, 2008, 2016; Ward, 2015).

Considering the multitude of ways bi+ experience can unfold, it is likely that bi+ lived experience is higher than reported – and highly likely to show up in the therapy room.

Health

Research consistently indicates that bi+ people have worse mental and physical health than gay, lesbian, and heterosexual people and that their health is impacted by challenges that are specifically related to their identity. Numerous studies indicate health disparities, including self-harm, suicidal ideation, substance use, sexual health, stress, eating disorders, anxiety, depression, and stress, for example (see Feinstein & Dyar, 2017; Habibi & Stueck, 2018; Barker et al., 2012; Movement Advancement Project, 2016 for an in-depth review).

Health care professionals are tasked with considering these findings within a biopsychosocial context, acknowledging the impact of wider social norms and cultural contexts (Barker, 2015), and how these may impact the daily lived experience of bi+ people. Bi+ minority stress is currently believed to be a key reason for these health disparities (Feinstein & Dyar, 2017).

Bi+ minority stress and double discrimination

Alongside the model of minority stress (see Meyer, 2003), understanding bi+ minority stress is facilitated by contextualising its position within both monosexism and heteronormativity – here defined by Eisner (2013):

> Monosexism is a social structure operating through the presumption that everyone is, or should be monosexual, a structure that privileges monosexuality and mono-sexual people, and that systemically punishes people who are nonmonosexual.
>
> (p. 63)

> Heteronormativity is a set of cultural and social norms, according to which there are only two binary genders (man and woman), and the only accept-able form of sexuality and romance is between one cisgender man and one cisgender woman. According to heteronormative standards, any lifestyle or behaviour deviating from the above is abnormal and should change to fit.
>
> (p. 47)

From this position, bi+ minority stress can be distinguished from gay and lesbian minority stress. It takes into account the prevalence of bi+ erasure in society and the 'double discrimination' (Ochs, 1996) and hostility faced by bi+ people from outside the wider LGBTQIA+ community and within it.

Biphobia (or bi+ phobia) refers to the unhelpful, negative, harmful, and stigma-tised ways that bi+ people are viewed; and can originate from external sources, as well as become internalised. Ochs (2021) represents this visually (adapted version is shown in Figure 6.1), outlining bi+ people's experience of external and inter-nalised homophobia and biphobia.

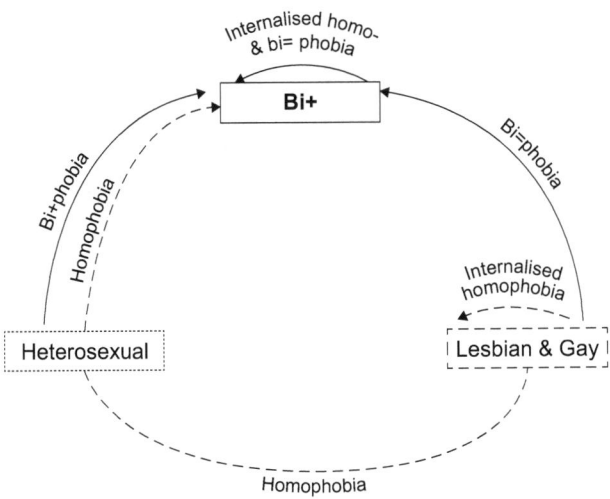

Figure 6.1 A visual representation of bi+ experiences of external and internalised homopho-bia and biphobia.

Biphobic views often highlight the perceived illegitimacy of bi+ identities, negative character traits, and partner unsuitability; and span denial, invisibility, marginalisation and exclusion, and stereotypes (Barker et al., 2012). Biphobia can be both explicit and felt more subtly. Barker (2016) acknowledges that for many, daily existence comes with extra emotional work. This echoes Turner's (2021) account of microaggressions:

> much like the death by 10,000 cuts, these are a form of psychological death. Yet . . . a microaggression is also a barely felt experience. It has a subtlety all of its own and is often different to spot in its aggressiveness and/or its deeper psychological impact.
>
> (p. 81)

Discussing sexual fluidity,Gawler-Wright (2016) notes that: 'non-static identity is experienced as unpredictable, unreliable, unstable, too complicated, unknowable, hidden' (5.38–5.51); and Bostwick and Hequembourg (2014) list bi+ specific microaggressions as hostility, denial/dismissal, unintelligibility, pressure to change, legitimacy, dating exclusion, and hypersexuality.

Intersectionality

Eliason and Elia (2011) caution simplistic thinking (or teaching) about bisexuality, suggesting that 'efforts that place all human sexual and social identities on intersecting continua that are socially and historically contingent will be much more useful in breaking down artificial binary positions' (p. 418).

Intersectionality offers a theory and framework for therapists to consider social inequality, power structures, and dynamics, and refrain from offering reductionist psychological and mental health formulations (Nayak, 2021). It 'enables a repositioning of shame and blame from the individual to the situations they inhabit' (Nayak, 2021, p. xxxiii).

Whilst therapists may be aware of the intersecting identities their clients hold (e.g. race, culture, class, age, gender, religion, disability, physical appearance, faith, and religion), working well with these can feel complex. Alongside bi+ minority stress, some clients will experience multiple discriminations due to multiple marginalised statuses. Lim and Hewitt (2018) note that 'intersectional theory offers a framework . . . premised on the idea that the structural oppressions are inter-locking and that multiple social identities interact with one another to produce unique social realities' (p. 322).

For example, bi+ trans and non-binary people may face double invisibility and discrimination; black bisexual women are objectified in relation to race, sexuality, and gender and face hypersexualisation (Barker et al., 2012); and bisexual men are seen as 'gay, gender non-conforming, hypersexual . . . vectors for the transmission of HIV and STIs' (Flanders, 2018, p. 138).

Bi+ erasure and invisibility

Bi+ erasure refers to the overt and covert erasure of bi+ experience, rendering it invisible (see Hayfield, 2021, for an in-depth review). McLean (2018) suggests three ways (see Table 6.2) bisexuality is missing from our sexual landscape: absence, appropriation, and assimilation.

Table 6.2 Three ways bisexuality is missing from our sexual landscape

Absence	External mechanism	• Bisexuality is absent from media, human rights campaigns, language, education, textbooks, and trainings.
Appropriation	External mechanism	• Many bisexual people are assigned a different identity (such as gay, lesbian, or heterosexual) often due to the gender of people they are in a relationship with. • Bisexuality is often subsumed under acronyms and words, such as LGBTQIA+ and queer.
Assimilation	Internal process	• Individuals may feel pressured to 'choose a side' or remain hidden for many reasons, including hostility and discrimination from many sides.

Identity debates and intra community minority stress

Sexual/romantic identities and the meanings clients ascribe to them can offer a sense of belonging and validity. Alongside this, there has been a rise of identity 'policing' in places like social media, which refers to debates about the 'right' meaning of particular labels. Whilst these conversations are important in wider contexts (academic and otherwise), when directed towards an individual about their lived experience, this can feel invalidating and destabilising. For example, Barker (2015) describes the experience: 'We bash up against each other, in conflict, leaving everyone feeling bruised, confused and betrayed, and perhaps reinforcing the ways in which we all criticize ourselves' (p. 380). Similarly, Feinstein et al. (2019) note that identity invalidation can lead to 'negative emotions, identity-related challenges, and relational difficulties' (p. 461).

Knowing that clients may arrive with a backlog of invalidating experiences is relevant both in terms of how cautious clients may feel about disclosing their identity, experiences, or attractions in therapy; as well as where therapists signpost clients to in the wider community.

Considering therapy with bi+ individuals

The therapist's role in perpetuating bi+ invisibility and accidental conversion therapy

Within the context of bi+ erasure and invisibility in education, many therapists may feel uneducated about the difficulties faced by bi+ people, which can impact therapy provided. At best, therapists who are unaware of bi+ experience may reinforce their client's experience of internalised bi-invisibility (D, 2018). At worst, therapists may be practising unintended conversion therapy.

For groups where invisibility is high, unintended conversion therapy may be more prevalent. A well-intentioned therapist who is uneducated about bi+ lived experience might assume their client is struggling to accept their 'real' monosexual identity and aim to support them to do so. Equally, a therapist with a limited understanding of bi+ lived experience might assume their client's identity is static and inflexible, instead of being aware of the multitude of individual experiences, sexual fluidity (occurring over time, or as an identity); or that for some, a bi+ label offers a valid stepping stone on their way to claiming a monosexual identity.

Pre-th erapy

Prospective clients may be looking for signs that a therapist is informed and affirmative about their struggles and concerns. Some therapists may choose to actively indicate that they work with bi+ clients as part of their marketing. Others may choose to disclose their own GSRD or bi+ identity (see Chapter 13).

Health care providers and bi+ experience

Many bi+ people have had negative experiences, and faced discrimination and invalidation from a variety of different health care providers, including therapists. This is important, not only in relation to a specific incident, but also because anti-bisexual experiences with mental health providers negatively impact the intent to reach out for future mental health support (see DeLucia & Smith for exploration of research, 2021). Bisexual people face barriers to healthcare; and once there, are less likely to share their orientation than gay and lesbian clients (Smalley et al., 2015). Whilst clients should not be pressured to disclose parts of their life they choose not to, identity concealment due to fear of discrimination or victimisation is associated with increased depression and generalised anxiety (Feinstein et al., 2020).

Therefore, therapists are encouraged to take an affirmative stance where diversity is valued and respected, and foster a safe enough space for clients to share themselves more fully if they wish to. Meeting each client in their unique lived experience also affords the opportunity to locate oppressive structures and norms within a society, and help lift any shame clients may feel for not managing to move forward alone. Additionally, it's important to acknowledge that for some, danger and harm related to orientation may be very real, both psychologically and physically; as is the unique stress of bi-invisibility, monosexism, and bi+ negativity/bi+ phobia.

Therapeutic relationship

Given that bi+ people often report feeling isolated and lonely (Page, 2004), the therapeutic relationship may hold particular importance. For some clients, working with a therapist who is respectful, kind, affirmative, and who offers a safer relational space may be a new experience. These experiences may evoke feelings of vulnerability, or emotions that do not feel familiar or initially safe. Attunement to pacing may be important, and it may take time to build trust within the alliance. For some clients, the therapist may be the first person who hasn't rushed them into claiming an identity, but instead has sat alongside them in their dilemmas and desires, at odds with dominant narratives around gender, sex, and relationships. D (2016) notes that clients experiencing internalised negative meanings about bisexuality often come to therapy with shame, confusion, isolation, guilt, fear about what their feelings mean, and experience bisexuality as a burden. Regardless of the model of therapy, such experiences will need to be attended to with care and attunement.

Language and identity

It is important to use the client's language and identities in therapy. Some clients may want to explore different labels, to 'try on' different identities, and think about what these evoke. The question 'what does this open up and what does this close down?' (Iantaffi & Barker, 2019) can be a helpful starting place: what ways of being in the world, what feelings, what experiences?

Speaking up

Given the prevalence of bi+ erasure, therapists may find that voicing an alternative normalising narrative is needed – both in terms of the existence of bi+ lived experience, and of living within a bi+ negative and erasing society. Depending on your preferred therapeutic model, this may, or may not, feel out of the ordinary.

Microaffirmations

Foregrounding the possibility of microaggressions at the start of therapy is one way of demonstrating that you are open and willing to receive feedback, and that therapy provides a safer space to bring up difficult relational moments. It may lead to more opportunities to work with rupture and repair, and the therapeutic benefits this can offer. If a client feels safe enough to share a microaggression with you, hearing their pain, accepting your role, and moving forward may offer the kind of 'working through' that hasn't previously been possible.

Microaffirmations (Rowe, 2008) can be defined as 'subtle interpersonal acts of support or validation that are often enacted unconsciously' (DeLucia & Smith, 2021, p. 146).

Although little research has looked at the experience of microaffirmations within the context of bi+ therapy, Flanders (2015) suggests that positive identity experiences can decrease stress and anxiety, and DeLucia and Smith (2021) suggest microaffirmations might look like: 'offering support or asking sincere questions about bisexuality' (p. 146). Given that clients will bring their own unique lived experiences to therapy, we can anticipate that microaffirmative experiences will shift accordingly. Research indicates that interpersonal relationships provide opportunities to experience microaffirmations (Flanders et al., 2017), and the therapeutic relationship offers a unique and potentially reparative relationship in this regard.

Considerations about myths, assumptions, and binary thinking

Eisner (2013) challenges bisexual myths and related assumptions. As we consider some of the stereotypes and myths around bi+ lived experience, it may feel tempting to take the opposite position. However, these positions may also feel unhelpful or limited, offering a 'counter myth' (see Table 6.3).

Table 6.3 Reconsidering and challenging bi+ myths, assumptions, and polarised positions

Myth	Assumption	Opposite position/ counter myth	Open/balanced view
Bisexuality is a phase	Phases are invalid	Bisexuality is static	It may be a phase/stage that lasts any amount of time (including all of life); life is a continual unfolding; all stages in life are valid
Bi+ people are promiscuous	Casual sex or sex with many people is 'bad'	Bi+ people don't have casual sex	Within the parameters of sexual health (World Health Organization, 2006), no amount, or way, of having sex is better or worse than another
Bi+ people are confused	Confusion = Invalid experience	Bi+ people don't feel confused, they are always certain of their identity	Having questions about ourselves and noticing confusion at times, ambivalence, or nuance as we grow can be normalised – it doesn't invalidate experience or identity, or mean it is a 'lesser' experience
Bi+ people can't be monogamous	Monogamy is best, preferred	Bi+ people are monogamous	There are lots of relationship structures available, none better or worse than any other

Whilst the myths in Table 6.3 correspond with stigmatised views of bi+ identities, the 'counter myths' could be seen as 'being good' or more in line with normative expectations.

Either polarised position forces the client into a tight box, with little space to lean into their authentic way of relating to others or themselves. When therapists honour diversity and remain open to the people in front of them, they can affirm their client's unique experiences, desires, and hopes for their life, and support them more fully. If clients are feeling pressure to be the 'poster child for the good bisexual', it can be useful to gently unpack why they might feel this pressure, and allow them to move towards a more balanced and open view.

Coming out and being in relationships

Research relating to coming out suggests experiences are varied for bi+ people – at times, even negatively impacting their mental health (Habibi & Stueck, 2018). It may be beneficial to foster a safe enough space to explore what the process may look like (often an ongoing process) and the variety of ways relationships may be impacted. Client safety is a key aspect of therapy. If clients are in intimate relationships, therapists should hold in mind the possibility and prevalence of intimate partner violence (IPV; see Chapter 8), as well as any bi+ phobic discrimination that clients may experience.

Narratives of resilience

Narratives of hope and resilience can be an important part of therapeutic endeavours. The mechanisms of bi+ erasure may mean that clients have not heard a narrative of visibility, joy, and resilience; and therapy may provide the opportunity for new meaning-making in relation to themselves and their place in the world. Research can help guide this. For example, Rostosky et al. (2010) outlined positive aspects of bisexuality; and where relevant, these can offer jumping-off points for client exploration (see Table 6.4).

Table 6.4 Positive aspects of bisexuality

Self	Freedom from social labels
	Honesty and authenticity
	Having a unique perspective
	Increased insight and awareness
Interpersonal relationships	Freedom to love without regard for sex/gender
	Freedom to explore relationships
	Freedom of sexual expression
Society and community	Acceptance of diversity
	Belonging to community
	Understanding privilege and oppression
	Becoming an advocate/activist

Other studies have indicated bisexual affirmative experiences happen at intra-personal, interpersonal, and institutional levels (Flanders et al., 2017). These include belonging to a community, normalisation, acceptance, visibility, providing or receiving support, talking about shared experiences, celebrating identity; and community, personal growth, and not feeling limited by gender (Wang & Feinstein, 2020). These may prompt ideas for reaching out to community and other relationships outside the therapy room.

Considering narrative, Gawler-Wright (2016) explores some qualities related to fluidity and identity, such as: 'truthful, open, flexible, brave, accepting, evolving, multi-layered' (6.24–6.41). Barker (2016) acknowledges the courage it can take to claim a bisexual identity and that as people who may have experienced both privilege and oppression (who can understand both these positions and what it is like to live within these spaces), bisexual people can be 'bridge builders' in society.

These narratives may also be available when considering intersectionality. For example, for trans and nonbinary people, rather than being seen as a burden or negatively framed, bisexuality can indicate a sexual identity that sits outside gender binaries (Langridge & Barker, 2016). Over time, the lived experience of older bisexual people may be a 'potential source of growth' (Sinnott, 2016, p. 3), and a narrative of 'positive intersectionality' can act as a possible factor of resilience for LGBTQ-POC (Ghabrial, 2017).

Regardless of the theoretical model used, drawing on research and literature may help guide clients towards a more positive self-narrative, and an opportunity to reflect on the affirmative experiences that they have had with others.

Opportunities and signposting

Gonzales et al. (2021) explore the importance of belonging and community connection for bi+ people, noting the need for welcoming and inclusive spaces. Many people find community spaces affirmative – whether this is queer-identified, bi+ specific, or another non-bi+ specific community. However, this is not uniform, and it is worth considering what benefits and challenges may arise, particularly in relation to intersectionality (Langridge & Barker, 2016).

Bi+ affirmative therapy does not always mean bi+ focused therapy

Many people with bi+ lived experience may feel content in their identity. They may have grown up around, or be part of, friendship groups, sexual/romantic relationships, family, and/or communities who are affirmative, informed, and supportive. You may meet clients who feel secure and settled in their desires, behaviours, attractions, and the various ways they want to have relationships with others, and reach out for therapy for unrelated reasons. For these clients, working with a bi+ aware therapist may reduce fear that a therapist will over-focus on sexual/romantic lived experience, sensationalise, fragilize, or victimise them. The most affirmative experience will be accepting their identity/lived experience whilst focusing on whatever has brought them to therapy.

Relationship therapy, where one partner has bi+ lived experience

The following section draws on literature regarding mixed-orientation relationships, however, much of what is written may be relevant to bi+ people in a relationship together as well. Relationship therapists hold space for all people in a relationship and can acknowledge the impact, regardless of orientation, that living in a heteronormative, monosexist society has. As well as holding in mind what this may be like for bi+ partners, therapists also hold in mind monosexual partners and their invisible experience in this context, which is often 'minimised or ignored' (Buxton, 2011, p. 539).

Dating

For the purpose of considering what clients may bring with them into mixed-orientation relationship therapy, a brief understanding of dating experiences can be helpful. For example, Feinstein and Dyar (2018) review literature regarding sexual and romantic relationships, noting that heterosexual people often view bisexual people as unacceptable partners; people expect to experience insecurity and jealousy with a bisexual partner; bisexual people are seen as more likely to pass on an STI to their partner (than gay, lesbian, and heterosexual people); and bisexual men are seen as less trustworthy, or less able to maintain a long-term relationship (see Feinstein & Dyar, 2018, for a full review).

Gender and orientation of partner

Research suggests that gender and orientation may intersect in unique ways in mixed-orientation relationships, although findings are not always consistent. For example, having a partner who is supportive of a bisexual identity can have a positive impact on well-being (Li et al., 2013) and act as a buffer against stress (Meyer, 2003). However, being in a mixed-orientation relationship has also been associated with increased anxiety symptoms (including social anxiety, generalised anxiety disorder, and posttraumatic stress disorder; Feinstein et al., 2016). Bisexual women in heterosexual passing relationships are shown to maintain relationship satisfaction (Reinhardt, 2001) but also may experience increased depression, alcohol use, and internalised binegativity (Molina et al., 2015). Bisexual women in same-sex relationships may experience increased uncertainty about their orientation (Dyar et al., 2014).

Being educated about bi+ lived experience and mixed-orientation relationships facilitates therapists' attunement to their clients. They are able to support their clients' hopes for therapy and refrain from centring all of the relationship's stuck points on bi+ lived experience. Whilst this chapter focuses primarily on research about bi+ people in dyads, bi+ people may be in relationships of any relationship structure (also see Chapters 1, 2, and 3).

Therapeutic relationship

A relationship therapist may be the only person to witness and be alongside their clients as they navigate relationship dilemmas, difficulties, and change. Clients may not know anyone else who has faced the dilemmas they have, and arrive feeling vulnerable, ashamed, uncertain, or thinking something is fundamentally flawed or 'wrong' with them or the relationship.

Therapists are in a unique position to offer a normalising, informed perspective, and provide a safe enough space to explore experiences and dilemmas. Building trust in the therapeutic relationship may take some time, and attunement to process, individually and together, will aid this. With empathy, congruence, respect, and attunement, therapists can tease out the specificities of dilemmas, validate each person, and be alongside the relationship as it unfolds and evolves. They can model holding seemingly opposing positions at the same time without becoming polarised. Alongside this, there may be times that interventions offer boundaries and limit hostility in ways that are both ethical and unknown within the relationship space, which can also increases feelings of safety.

Assessment and therapeutic frameworks

Whilst theoretical models guide the approach to assessment, Crofford (2018) offers guidance that practitioners may find helpful. Although written with dyads in mind, much is relevant to other relationship structures. The assessment may include individual sessions with both the bi+ partner and non-bi+ partner, and joint sessions. Depending on the model of therapy used, how this looks may vary (see Table 6.5).

Table 6.5 Considerations for the assessment phase of therapy

Individual session with bi+ partner	Identity/orientation, experiences of binegativity/related trauma, community connection, identity maintenance.
Individual session with non-bi+ partner	Identity/orientation, feelings about bisexuality and partner identity, whether this is shared with friends and family, and how their partner disclosed their identity.
Joint session	Revisiting incongruences within the relationship; experiences of binegativity; defining what commitment means within their relationship; and dealing with invisibility and discrimination.

It may also be helpful to include specific inventories such as the 'bisexual identity inventory', and 'attitudes regarding bisexuality scale'; as well as assessing mental health, IPV, sexual health, and experiences related to the relationship (such as of parenting/pregnancy, for example; Crofford, 2018). In keeping with this book as a whole, as mixed-orientation relationship therapy continues, you are encouraged to use a GSRD aware and affirmative approach. You may also wish to consider the ex-PLISSIT model (Taylor & Davis, 2007) and consider appropriate referral sources where relevant.

Dilemmas in the room

Crofford (2018) summarises some of the reasons that people in mixed-orientation relationships may come to therapy: 'negotiating commitment and coming out as bisexual or otherwise same-sex attracted . . . and challenges related to parenting, communication, intimacy, or even separating amicably' (p. 234).

In order to bring some dilemmas to life, client vignettes follow, posing certain questions: where are the more general relationship themes, and where does a dilemma seem specific to bi+ experience? These dilemmas are often nuanced. Making these kinds of discernments in therapy helps to refrain from problematising bi+ experience itself, or losing the opportunity to normalise bi+ experience within diversity as a whole.

Liz and Johan

Liz and Johan have dated for 6 months. Liz has been out as pansexual for 5 years, and her last relationship was with a woman. Her social circle was mainly orientated within the lesbian community and spaces. Since they started dating, Liz doesn't feel welcome in the predominantly femme/lesbian friendship groups or spaces. She is grieving multiple losses, and her mood is low. Some of her friends have distanced themselves from her since she started dating a man. Johan identifies as straight and, as far as he is aware, has not been in a mixed-orientation relationship before. He feels helpless, angry with Liz's friends, and like he is in a situation he doesn't fully understand. Some of his friends have mentioned they are concerned he's going to get hurt given that 'she'll probably go back to women at some point'. Johan has become Liz's main source of connection, which is making them both feel uneasy in different ways.

Raj and Tim

Raj and Tim are in a non-monogamous relationship. Raj identifies as gay, and his activist identity is important to him. He has never considered himself biphobic and didn't think Tim's bi identity would bother him when they started dating. Over the last few months, he has noticed that whilst he feels fine about Tim having sex with other men, he is worried when Tim has sex with people of other genders. He says he's concerned that Tim will leave him for someone of a different gender. He feels ashamed that he is anxious, and knows Tim has given him no reason to doubt how satisfied he is in the relationship. He feels like his activist identity is threatened by his unfounded fears about bisexuality and wishes he could 'get over them'. He feels the urge to constantly ask for reassurance. Initially, Tim found this connecting and enjoyed offering reassuring words and comforting touch, but more recently he now feels untrusted.

Tom and Clare

Tom has been out as sexually fluid and queer in most areas of his life for many years. He and Clare (who doesn't label herself, but is attracted to people rather than gender) are primary partners in a poly relationship. Family is important to them both; however, Clare is not open with her family about either her sexuality or being in a poly relationship, and does not want Tom to come out to them. She knows her family hold homophobic beliefs and doesn't want them to view Tom or her differently. She wishes Tom could 'let it go'. Tom has started to feel uneasy and is refusing to visit Clare's family if he has to 'monitor himself all the time'. They both feel frustrated with the other and have started to argue, feeling unsure about their future.

Sabine and Alban

Sabine and Alban are a heterosexual-identifying couple who have been together for 20+ years. Sabine recently told Alban she has erotic fantasies about people she climbs with, noting that trusting someone with her life threads throughout her fantasies. Alban was surprised. He wanted to turn to friends to talk, but they are joint friends, and Sabine did not want to be 'gossiped about'. Alban says he feels isolated – he hasn't heard about this happening to anyone else in a long-term relationship. He explains Sabine's disclosure has brought up questions about his own attractions in ways he hadn't previously considered. Sabine had been hoping to lean on Alban for support, but she feels disappointed by how their conversations have gone, and wishes she didn't feel the attractions she does.

The breakdown in Table 6.6 presents bi+ specific and more general relationship themes.

Having read through the vignettes, what else might you add?

Table 6.6 Client vignettes: bi+ specific and general relationship themes

Bi+ specific	General
Bi+ lived experience	Secrecy and withholding
Internalised bi+ phobia	Fear of others' judgements about past
Fears of being 'outed'	What of ourselves do we share vs keep
The choice to keep identity private	private in different circles?
Feeling silenced by partner	Evolving self over time
Longing for another gender	Missed communication (assumptions about
Bi+ experience is a burden	partner's thoughts being made)
Pulled between being out/'passing'	The fluidity of attractions in various ways
Ongoing considerations about	over a lifetime
coming out	Shared friendships and relationship issues
	Different ways of relating to biological
Partner	family than a partner
Fear of homophobia/bi+ phobia	Conflict/disagreement
from others	Longing for what is outside the
Bi+ phobia as unexpected	relationship
Internalised biphobia: self-doubt and	Loss of the sense you had of the other
shame	Navigating societal norms and cultural
Starting to think more broadly	expectations
about attraction	Intersectionality
Impact of societal bi+ erasure on	Mental health
relationship anxiety felt	Impact of the timing of disclosures
Resentment that partner isn't	Guilt and shame
content 'passing' in a monosexual or	Trust
normative way	Boundaries
	Communication

Here are a few considerations that may be particularly relevant for people in mixed-orientation relationships.

Timing of disclosure

Moments of relational crisis may be accompanied by unexpected disclosure (of many kinds). Disclosure can signify a shift in the relationship, where someone finds out they are in a relationship that they didn't consent to be part of. This may or may not be relevant for the clients that you meet who are in mixed-orientation relationships. Many may enter into the relationship already knowing the bi+ orientation of their partner. Where bi+ disclosure happens some years into the relationship, Buxton (2006) notes that it may take some time to process what this means for the relationship and individuals within it. Therapists who are educated about bi+ lived experience and mixed-orientation relationships are in a unique position to offer affirmative therapeutic support to their clients as these conversations unfold.

Relationship structures

Consensual non-monogamy (CNM) and monogamy may offer bi+ people different possibilities: polyamorous relationships may offer inclusivity and feel bi+ affirmative, yet add to bi+ stereotypes; whilst monogamy may provide emotional and psychological benefits of being in a couple, but create difficulty in regards to visibility and self-identity (Robinson, 2013). Bi+ individuals are often assumed to be heterosexual, gay, or lesbian in relationships, depending on the gender of their partner. The impact of this on a non-monosexual person can be part of a daily emotional burden: the psychological stress of self-erasure and the impact on the person's sense of self, agency, and belonging; as well as engaging in ongoing decisions about whether to repeatedly come out or not. People in mixed-orientation relationships may work together to reimagine and redesign what monogamy means to them, consider practising gendered monogamy (Pallotta-Chiarolli, 2014), or explore different relationship structures (see Chapters 1, 2, and 3).

Abuse and power

Whilst the earlier vignettes aim to offer insight into dilemmas that are nuanced, it is also important to highlight concerns related to power and abuse. Bisexual men and women face an increased risk of IPV victimisation compared to monosexual people (Walters et al., 2013). Habibi and Stueck (2018) collate research that particularly indicates the negative experiences and impact on bisexual women; and more recently, Chen et al. (2020) found that bisexual women experience more stalking, IPV, and IPV-related impact than heterosexual women and lesbians, and more contact sexual violence (CSV) than lesbians. Feinstein and Dyar (2018) reflect that one possible reason for increased IPV may be a monosexual partner's concerns, jealousy, and insecurity. Power and abuse may show up in both overt and covert ways, and within the context of bi+ experience could include some of the following: shaming, name-calling, trivialising, banning, coercion into sexual situations, and being in situations that are not consented to (D, 2016). Awareness of the possibility of abuse and power dynamics within the larger context of heteronormativity, monosexism, and intersectionality (as well as your own position within these contexts) is vital. These findings may also impact therapeutic exploration regarding disclosure (see Chapter 8).

Concluding

Having considered both individual and relationship therapy with bi+ people, and the wider context of bi+ lived experience, as we conclude, you are invited to reflect on the following questions. You may also wish to take these to supervision and explore further; and some further resources are detailed at the end.

Questions and reflections for therapists

- What assumptions do I hold about bi+ lived experience and identities?
- What gaps in knowledge do I have, and where can I educate myself?

- How can I challenge my own internalised bi+ negativity?
- Can I allow myself to connect to the oppression experienced and awaken compassion?
- How do I use language verbally and in written material: is it inclusive?
- How do I understand my own sexuality?
- Where can I access specialist supervision?
- What other bi+ aware service providers or community settings can I signpost clients to?
- Given microaggressions occur in therapy, how can I ensure I let the client know it's safe to bring these up with me?
- What do I understand as anti-oppressive therapy?
- What is my part to play in challenging bi+ erasure and bi+ phobia in society?
- If I identify as bi+, how can I ensure I practise self-care in the face of biphobia in the therapy room and de-centre myself so that I don't over-identify with a bi+ client?

Resources

Eisner, S. (2013). *Bi: Notes for a Bisexual Revolution.* Berkeley, CA. Seal Press.
Harrad, K. (Ed.). (2016). *Purple Prose: Bisexuality in Britain.* Portland: Thorntree Press.
https://bicommunitynews.co.uk/
https://biresource.org/
https://stillbisexual.com/
Iantaffi, A., & Barker, M.-J. (2019). *Life Isn't Binary: On Being Both, Beyond, and in-Between.* London: Jessica Kingsley Publishers.
www.bisexualindex.org.uk/

References

Barker, M.-J. (2015). Depression and/or oppression? Bisexuality and mental health. *Journal of Bisexuality, 15*(3), 369–384.
Barker, M.-J. (2016). *Pink Therapy Conference: 'Bisexuality and Mental Health'.* Retrieved from www.youtube.com/watch?v=9aXd-ihLjiY
Barker, M., Richards, C., Jones, R., Bowes-Catton, H., Plowman, T., Yockney, J., & Morgan, M. (2012). *The Bisexuality Report: Bisexual Inclusion in LGBT Equality and Diversity.* Centre for Citizenship, Identity and Governance. The Open University. Retrieved from http://oro.open.ac.uk/52881/1/The%20BisexualityReport%20Feb.2012_0.pdf
Bostwick, W., & Hequembourg, A. (2014). 'Just a little hint': Bisexual-specific microaggressions and their connection to epistemic injustices. *Culture, Health and Sexuality, 16*, 488–503.
Buxton, A. P. (2006). Counseling heterosexual spouses of bisexual men and women and bisexual-heterosexual couples. *Journal of Bisexuality, 6*(1–2), 105–135. http://doi.org/10.1300/J159v06n01_07
Buxton, A. P. (2011). Reflections on bisexuality through the prism of mixed-orientation marriages. *Journal of Bisexuality, 11*(4), 525–544. http://doi.org/10.1080/15299716.2011.620864

Chen, J., Walters, M. L., Gilbert, L. K., & Patel, N. (2020). Sexual violence, stalking, and intimate partner violence by sexual orientation, United States. *Psychology of Violence*, *10*(1), 110–119. https://doi.org/10.1037/vio0000252

Crofford, M. (2018). Bisexual inclusive couples therapy: Assessment and treatment with bisexuals in mixed orientation relationships. *Journal of Sexual and Relationship Therapy*, *33*(01–02). http://doi.org/10.1080/14681994.2017.1412420

D, N. (2016). *Pink Therapy Conference: Addressing Biphobia in Relationship Therapy.* Retrieved from www.youtube.com/watch?v=nhHoHffiP2A&list=PLjFNIE-UDKEnuctl-ZqCZAyoNwq9v84i3&index=8

D, N. (2018). Now you see me, now you don't: Addressing bisexual invisibility in relationship therapy. *Journal of Sexual and Relationship Therapy*, *33*(01–02).

Dahlgreen, W., & Shakespeare, A.-E. (2015). *YouGov: 1 in 2 Young People Say They Are Not 100% Heterosexual.* Retrieved from https://yougov.co.uk/topics/lifestyle/articles-reports/2015/08/16/half-young-not-heterosexual

DeLucia, R., & Smith, N. G. (2021). The impact of provider biphobia and microaffirmations on bisexual individuals' treatment-seeking intentions. *Journal of Bisexuality*, *21*(2), 145–166.

Diamond, L. M. (2008). *Sexual Fluidity: Understanding Women's Love and Desire.* Cambridge, MA: Harvard University Press.

Diamond, L. M. (2016). Sexual fluidity in male and females. *Current Sexual Health Reports*, *8*, 249–256.

Dyar, C., Feinstein, B. A., & London, B. (2014). Dimensions of sexual identity and minority stress among bisexual women: The role of partner gender. *Psychology of Sexual Orientation and Gender Diversity*, *1*(4), 441–451. http://doi.org/10.1037/sgd0000063

Eisner, S. (2013). *Bi: Notes for a Bisexual Revolution.* Berkeley, CA: Seal Press.

Eliason, M., & Elia, J. (2011). Reflections about bisexuality and the Journal of Bisexuality. *Journal of Bisexuality*, *11*, 412–419. http://doi.org/10.1080/15299716.2011.620463

Feinstein, B. A., & Dyar, C. (2017). Bisexuality, minority stress, and health. *Current Sexual Health Reports*, *9*(1), 42–49. http://doi.org/10.1007/s11930-017-0096-3

Feinstein, B. A., & Dyar, C. (2018). Romantic and sexual relationship experiences among bisexual individuals. In D. J. Swan & S. Habibi (Eds.), *Bisexuality: Theories, Research and Recommendations for the Invisible Sexuality* (pp. 145–163). Switzerland: Springer.

Feinstein, B. A., Franco, M., Henderson, R. F., Collins, L. K., & Davari, J. (2019). A qualitative examination of bisexual identity invalidation and its consequences for wellbeing, identity, and relationships. *Journal of Bisexuality*, *19*(4), 461–482.

Feinstein, B. A., Hall, C. D. X., Dyar, C., & Davila, J. (2020). Motivations for sexual identity concealment and their associations with mental health among bisexual, pansexual, queer, and fluid (Bi+) individuals. *Journal of Bisexuality*, *20*(3), 324–341. http://doi.org/10.1080/15299716.2020.1743402

Feinstein, B. A., Latack, J. A., Bhatia, V., Davila, J., & Eaton, N. R. (2016). Romantic relationship involvement as a minority stress buffer in gay/lesbian versus bisexual individuals. *Journal of Gay and Lesbian Mental Health*, *20*(3), 237–257. http://doi.org/10.1080/19359705.2016.1147401

Flanders, C. E. (2015). Bisexual health: A daily diary analysis of stress and anxiety. *Basic and Applied Social Psychology*, *37*(6), 319–335. http://doi.org/10.1080/01973533.2015.1079202

Flanders, C. E. (2018). The male bisexual experience. In D. J. Swan & S. Habibi (Eds.), *Bisexuality: Theories, Research and Recommendations for the Invisible Sexuality* (pp. 127–143). Switzerland: Springer.

Flanders, C. E., Tarasoff, L. A., Legge, M. M., Robinson, M., & Gos, G. (2017). Positive identity experiences of young bisexual and other nonmonosexual people: A qualitative inquiry. *Journal of Homosexuality*, *64*(8), 1014–1032. http://doi.org/10.1080/00918369 .2016.1236592

Galupo, M. P. (2018). Plurisexual identity labels and the marking of bisexual desire. In D. J. Swan & S. Habibi (Eds.), *Bisexuality: Theories, Research and Recommendations for the Invisible Sexuality* (pp. 61–75). Switzerland: Springer.

Gawler-Wright, P. (2016). *Pink Therapy Conference: 'Three Dirty Words: Choice. Confusion. Fluidity'*. Retrieved from www.youtube.com/watch?v=f4Ktp6jU9wQ

Ghabrial, M. A. (2017). "Trying to figure out where we belong": Narratives of racialized sexual minorities on community, identity, discrimination, and health. *Sexuality Research and Social Policy: A Journal of the NSRC*, *14*(1), 42–55. https://doi.org/10.1007/ s13178-016-0229-x

Gonzalez, A., Flanders, C. E., Pulice-Farrow, L., & Bartnik, A. (2021). "It's almost like bis, pans kind of stick together:" Bi+Belonging and community connection. *Journal of Bisexuality*, *21*(2), 194–224. http://doi.org/10.1080/15299716.2021.1927282

Habibi, S., & Stueck, F. (2018). Well-being: Bisexuality and mental and physical health. In D. J. Swan & S. Habibi (Eds.), *Bisexuality: Theories, Research and Recommendations for the Invisible Sexuality* (pp. 165–188). Switzerland: Springer.

Hayfield, N. (2021). *Bisexual and Pansexual Identities: Exploring and Challenging Invisibility and Invalidation*. Oxon: Routledge.

Iantaffi, A., & Barker, M.-J. (2019). *Life Isn't Binary: On Being Both, Beyond, and in-Between*. London: Jessica Kingsley Publishers.

Klein, F. (1993). *The Bisexual Option: Second Edition*. The American Institute of Bisexuality, Inc.

Langridge, F., & Barker, M.-J. (2016). The gender agender. In K. Harrad (Ed.), *Purple Prose: Bisexuality in Britain*. Portland: Thorntree Press.

Li, T., Dobinson, C., Scheim, A. I., & Ross, L. E. (2013). Unique issues bisexual people face in intimate relationships: A descriptive exploration of lived experience. *Journal of Gay and Lesbian Mental Health*, *17*(1), 21–39. http://doi.org/10.1080/19359705.2012. 723607

Lim, G., & Hewitt, B. (2018). Discrimination at the intersections: Experiences of community and belonging in nonmonosexual persons of color. *Journal of Bisexuality*, *18*(3), 318–352. http://doi.org/10.1080/15299716.2018.1518182

McLean, K. (2018). Bisexuality in society. In D. J. Swan & S. Habibi (Eds.), *Bisexuality: Theories, Research and Recommendations for the Invisible Sexuality* (pp. 77–93). Switzerland: Springer.

Meyer, I. H. (2003). Prejudice, social stress, and mental health in lesbian, gay and bisexual populations: Conceptual issues and research evidence. *Psychological Bulletin*, *129*, 674–697. http://doi.org/10.1037/0033-2909.129.5.674

Molina, Y., Marquez, J. H., Logan, D. E., Leeson, C. J., Balsam, K. F., & Kaysen, D. L. (2015). Current intimate relationship status, depression, and alcohol use among bisexual women: The mediating roles of bisexual-specific minority stressors. *Sex Roles*, *73*(1), 43–57. https://doi.org/10.1007/s11199-015-0483-z

Movement Advancement Project. (2016, September). *Invisible Majority: The Disparities Facing Bisexual People and How to Remedy Them*. Retrieved September 4, 2021, from www.lgbtmap.org/policy-and-issue-analysis/invisible-majority

Nayak, S. (2021). Intersectionality and psychotherapy with an eye to clinical and professional ethics. In M. Trachsel, J. Gaab, N. Biller-Andorno, S. Tekin, & J. Z. Sadler

(Eds.), *The Oxford Handbook of Psychotherapy Ethics* (pp. 890–903). Oxford: Oxford University Press.

Ochs, R. (1996). Biphobia: It goes more than two ways. In B. A. Firestein (Ed.), *Bisexuality: The Psychology and Politics of an Invisible Minority* (pp. 217–239). Thousand Oaks: Sage.

Ochs, R. [@robynochs]. (2021, May 14). [photograph of graphic titled 'How both biphobia and homophobia affect bi+ people]. Retrieved from https://www.instagram.com/p/CO1 PridsGxn/?igshid=MDJmNzVkMjY=

Page, E. H. (2004). Mental health services experiences of bisexual women and bisexual men. *Journal of Bisexuality*, *4*(1–2), 137–160. http://doi.org/10.1300/J159v04n01_11

Pallotta-Chiarolli, M. (2014). New rules, no rules, old rules or our rules: Women designing mixedorientation relationships with bisexual men. In M. Pallotta-Chiarolli & B. Pease (Eds.), *The politics of recognition and social justice: Transforming subjectivities and new forms of resistance* (pp. 99–106). New York: Routledge.

Reinhardt, R. V. (2001). Bisexual women in heterosexual relationships. *Journal of Bisexuality*, *2*(2–3), 163–171. http://doi.org/10.1300/J159v02n02_11

Robinson, M. (2013). Polyamory and monogamy as strategic identities. *Journal of Bisexuality*, *13*(1), 21–38. http://doi.org/10.1080/15299716.2013.755731

Rostosky, S., Riggle, E., Pascale-Hague, D., & McCants, L. (2010). The positive aspects of a bisexual identification. *Psychology and Sexuality*, *1*, 131–144.

Rowe, M. (2008). Micro-affirmations and micro-inequities. *Journal of the International Ombudsman Association*, *1*, 45–48.

Sinnott, J. (2016). Introduction to the special issue on aging and bisexuality: Can these complex life patterns be an impetus for identity flexibility and growth? *Journal of Bisexuality*, *16*, 1–17. http://doi.org/10.1080/15299716.2016.1145992

Smalley, K. B., Warren, J. C., & Barefoot, K. N. (2015.) Barriers to care and psychological distress differences between bisexual and gay men and women. *Journal of Bisexuality*, *15*(2), 230–247. http://doi.org/10.1080/15299716.2015.1025176

Swan, D. J. (2018). Models and measures of sexual orientation. In D. J. Swan & S. Habibi (Eds.), *Bisexuality: Theories, Research and Recommendations for the Invisible Sexuality* (pp. 19–36). Switzerland: Springer.

Taylor, B., & Davis, S. (2007). The extended PLISSIT model for addressing the sexual wellbeing of individuals with an acquired disability or chronic illness. *Sexuality and Disability*, *25*, 135–139. http://doi.org/10.1007/s11195-007-9044-x

Turner, D. (2021). *Intersections of Privilege and Otherness in Counselling and Psychotherapy*. London: Routledge.

Walters, M. L., Chen, J., & Breiding, M. J. (2013). *The National Intimate Partner and Sexual Violence Survey (NISVS): 2010 Findings on Victimization by Sexual Orientation*. Atlanta: National Center for Injury Prevention and Control, Centers for Disease Control and Prevention.

Wang, A. Y., & Feinstein, B. A. (2020). The perks of being bi+: Positive sexual orientation – related experiences among bisexual, pansexual, and queer male youth. *Psychology of Sexual Orientation and Gender Diversity*. Advance online publication. https://doi.org/10.1037/sgd0000459

Ward, J. (2015). *Not Gay: Sex between Straight White Men*. New York: NYU Press.

World Health Organization. (2006). *Defining Sexual Health: Report of a Technical Consultation on Sexual Health 28–31 January 2002* (pp. 1–35). Geneva, Switzerland: WHO.

Chapter 7

Sankofa's Quest: Cultivating Queer, African-centred, homecomings through intersectionality in therapy

Joel Simpson

Sankofa, in Twi (a dialect of the Akan language of Ghana), translates loosely as return (san), go (ko), take (fa). Symbolically, Akan people capture Sankofa through a Bono Adinkra image: a mythical bird is depicted with a backwards-facing head, having retrieved a valuable egg in its mouth, and forward-facing feet (Willis, 1998). In the context of therapy with queer African diasporan people, Sankofa's quest encapsulates clients' unconscious and conscious longings for homecomings and the necessity of returning to our roots to retrieve, redeem, and ingest what may be of value from the past. Individuals and collectives may then claim and reclaim their potential and inheritance as they consider what they are being drawn towards and who they are becoming.

Whilst homecomings might be understood as reunions and returns from having departed and arrived back home, they can also evoke pain and disorientation when roots, customs, history and discourse have been severed, denied, and forgotten. The violent imposition of colonialism, religious-infused dogma, legislation and policies that govern civil liberties in relation to gender, relationships, and sexual diversity have denied many queer African-diasporan people the freedom to engage with wholly African ways of being. At the time of writing, around half of the sixty-eight countries worldwide that continue to criminalise homosexuality are former members of the British Empire and commonwealth members. The impact of imperialism in the UK, and across the globe, continues to threaten the potential of homecomings for queer African diasporan people. In these contexts, where and how might queer African diasporan clients return home to anchor, restore, and align with who they have been, might be, and are becoming?

In considering the cultivation of queer, African-centred homecomings and therapy through intersectionality, this chapter supports therapists to consider the necessity of integrating African-centred perspectives, such as Sankofa, within psychotherapeutic discourse and practice. The terms 'African diasporan' and 'queer' are explored. Conceptions of intersectionality as a 'verb' (Cho et al., 2013; May, 2015), rather than a noun, and its potential for social-justice–oriented therapy is contemplated. An overview of the impact of the legacies of the African Holocaust

DOI: 10.4324/9781003260561-8

and enslavement broadens discussions around racialised trauma. Colonial notions of gender, relationship, and sexual diversity are questioned. Based on composites of real experiences, a fictional client vignette, of working with Nyumbani-Kuja, is offered. This chapter offers a practical contextualisation of working soulfully with intersectionality, dreams, loss, despair, homelessness, suicide, and suicidal ideation, in the process of cultivating queer African diasporan homecomings. Final contemplations consider how therapists might cultivate their practices to support queer, African diasporans through Sankofa's quest.

The necessity of Sankofa and reclaiming African-centred discourse

Homecomings are critical for queer African diasporan people because the impact of having ingested Eurocentric ideology, through its many guises, and being robbed of their own ancestral indigenous wisdom has often led to a profound sense of loss and self-hatred. Like Sankofa's mythical bird image, homecomings allow queer African diasporan people to return to their roots to redeem 'new de-colonised eggs', so they may engage with their potential. Psycho-spiritual re-education and therapy are often necessary for this. African diasporan-centred queer history and discourse has been marginalised by European historicity, which is often advanced as universally applicable, true, and insufficiently questioned. Social justice necessitates liberating all that has been shackled into monocultural discourses and has wrongly made African-centred ways of being and knowing seem inferior. Such discourse has led to queer African diasporans feeling 'dislocated' (Mazama, 2017, p. 65): living in states of spiritual, cultural, and mental exile as a result of European cultural, intellectual, and psychological imperialism (ibid.).

Whilst therapy in the Global North can, in some contexts, often reflect the values and assumptions of its origins, therapists cultivating homecomings with queer African diasporan people are challenged to re-orient therapy from Eurocentrism to integrate African-centred historiographies and language that counters colonially imposed queerphobia. This chapter responds to gaps in psychotherapeutic literature that marginalises queer, African-centred perspectives. This chapter reclaims intellectual and experiential customs of including 'critical intersectional discourse' (Allen, 2012, p. 218) and the knowledge, imaginations, and histories of queer, African diasporan people. Sankofa's quest highlights the necessity of reclamation and continual returns to wholeness because 'Africanness' has experienced types of intellectual, cultural, and historical 'genocide' (Diop, 1991, pp. 1–2), resulting in perpetual displacement for many. Therapists ought not to misconstrue Sankofa's quest as 'nostalgia' – it is 'a form of counter-memory that reads existing archives and historical narratives against the grain – unpacking assumptions, noting gaps, and questioning official versions of events' (May, 2015, p. 54). This chapter permeates beyond disciplinary boundaries to expand the remit of psychotherapeutic literature, staying conscious of ignorance, bias, and stagnation.

African diasporan and Queer?

Many queer people of African diasporan heritage use 'black' to describe their racialised identity. Unrelated to skin colour, 'black' sometimes refers to 'a political positioning as a result of imperialism and racism' (Collins, 2000, p. 85). 'Black' clusters allyship and political identities for (B)black African, South Asian, and Caribbean experiences of colonial rule (Collins & Bilge, 2020, p. 85). However, such clustering doesn't substantially capture nuanced experiences of each groups' colonial domination – muddling historicity. This chapter purposefully resists using 'BME', 'BAME', 'POC', and 'black'; these are often constructions of whiteness, designated to African bodies as categories of identity that are often used without sufficient thought – further cementing the power of white-bodied European's colonising (Akomolafe, 2017b). Originally, Africans did not refer to themselves as black because they were without comparisons (Akomolafe, 2017a). Respect for idiosyncrasies that relate to ancestral lineage, history, and culture (Johnson & Henderson, 2005) must include the transgenerational impact of the African Holocaust with the recognition that historicity pre-dates colonialism and enslavement.

Despite intentions of resisting clustering experiences, notions of African-centred queerness have the potential to essentialise, universalise, and assume homogeneity. It is critical that therapy provides a suitable container for queer African diasporan clients to reclaim an aspect of being that has been denied. Queerness ought not to be misconstrued as an unconscious fixing of parameters, which omits cultural connotations and ambiguities, distinctness, oppression, and power dynamics, rendering groups invisible (Tamale, 2011). Generally conceived as patronymic to whiteness, objections to African-centred queerness are sometimes contested as a continuation of forging African realities and experiences into Eurocentric concepts (Allen, 2012). It could be reasonable to resist invitations to reclaim something that historically hasn't been constructed as inherently African (ibid.) as, for many, queerness often 'displaces and rarely addresses the concerns of African diasporan people' (Johnson, 2005, p. 128).

Yet still, recognising the plausibility of its polemics, including and going beyond slurs and the vernacular, 'queer' might provide scope to capture and 'oppose patriarchal heterosexist heteronormative binary configurations of sexual orientations and gender identities' (Nyanzi, 2014, p. 61). African-centred queerness may be considered as playful, inclusive, and expansive, rather than cementing identities (Johnson, 2005) and constraining how identities are conceived (ibid.). African-centred queerness is purposefully elusive, complementing its 'epistemologic and political agenda' (Belkin, 2020, p. 9). It 'deconstructs and debunks one-sided, monolithic definitions of who' (ibid.) African diasporan people may be. African-centred queerness is self-definitive (Nyanzi, 2014) which is advantageous for a people whose identity has been imposed. African-centred queerness allows for complex, nuanced, dynamic, non-static potential (Muñoz, 2009), alongside 'the possibility of change, movement, redefinition, and subversive performance – from year to year, from partner to partner, from day to day, and even from act to act' (Cohen, 2005, p. 23). African-centred queerness symbolises resilience, liberation, pride, and triumph for having survived oppression at the intersection of ancestral lineage, gender, sexuality, and relationship diversity (ibid., p. 24).

Intersectionality: a verb

Whilst intersectionality may be difficult to define, it may be conceived as a call for therapists to consider clients' ancestral lineage, 'class, gender, sexuality, class, nation, ability, ethnicity, and age – among others – as interrelated and mutually shaping one another' (Collins & Bilge, 2020, p. 2). Where these aspects of 'being' intersect, power relations (whether explicit, indiscernible, or implicit) constellate, evoke, maintain, and/or deny privilege, access, and social inequality that influence social relations in therapy. This is reflective of the diverse societies that client and therapist are a part of, alongside their own individual experiences of daily life (ibid.). When issues of dominance, privilege, agency, and oppression emerge through the clients' presentation and the therapeutic relationship, intersectionality invites therapists to engage actively to address social injustice (das Nair & Butler, 2012). In this way, following Crenshaw (2011), therapists are encouraged to consider intersectionality as a 'verb' (May, 2015, p. 19), this means considering 'what it *does* or *can do*' (May, 2015, p. 19) to a client and the clinical relationship, rather than relating to its 'definitional status as a noun' (ibid.).

Intersectionality as a verb elicits a dynamic psychotherapeutic response of engaging with problems and being curious about their incompleteness, rather than following steps and techniques – thus ignoring what intersectionality is actually doing or could do for the client and the therapeutic relationship. Engaging with intersectionality might evoke overwhelming emotions when trying to consider the complexities of subordination and domination, at differing times, and locations, and the ways social identities intersect and situate individuals (Romero, 2018). Yet, mastering understanding isn't the intention. Instead, intersectionality as a verb invites a collaborative meaning-making endeavour. The 'doing' of intersectionality is engaged through deconstructing how clients and therapists experience privilege and oppression at varying intersections of their simultaneous identities as an ongoing means of transforming social inequality and promoting social justice. The paradox of intersectionality is therapists are often invited to *do* by *not doing*. In practice, this means bearing with not knowing; allowing for the challenge of an unfolding and being without coherent links to act upon. Recognising the centrality of uncertainty in therapy, intersectionality invites therapists to work with ambiguity and complexity without rigidity. Rather than coherent, completed applicable frameworks, intersectionality is consistently 'under construction' (Collins & Bilge, 2020, p. 37), whilst being simultaneously deconstructed. Therapy that incorporates intersectionality is purposefully 'open-ended, dynamic, and "biased" toward realizing collective justice' (May, 2015, p. 251). It acknowledges that there are no quick fixes – which is a challenge to egoic/(s)heroic ways of being. It does 'not (and cannot) provide a magic bullet, or offer a "panacea" ' (ibid.; Bailey, 2010, p. 53). Instead, intersectionality recognises how subtlety and nuances, in relation to power, tend to lurk within hidden dynamics of relationships. As such, drawing on May (2015), practically, therapists might consider key questions: what is left out of what clients share/don't share about power? Which aspects of identities are omitted and included, and what's the impact of this on the therapeutic relationship and the individuals? How might the responses to these baseline questions be made meaning of in collaboration with clients? What might the social justice and transformative implications be when these questions are interrogated?

Intersectionality for therapists

Intersectionality calls for therapists to consider how their own thoughts and clinical interventions might perpetuate clients' subordination and privilege (Collins, 2000). Supervision can be helpful to consider how to address these conscious and unconscious dynamics in service of the work – at a pace clients can digest. Therapists perpetuate inequality by refusing, or being too scared, to address social injustice issues within the therapeutic relationship. Feelings of 'not knowing how' and 'being afraid' are often part of the constellated relational field between client and therapist, as well as the therapist's own complexes, which must be attended to. As a 'polyglot' (Collins et al., 2020, p. x), intersectionality's language invites therapists to actively address power and prejudice in clients' lives and therapeutic relationships. Within any given moment of a session, as a therapist, I may be dominant, complicit, vulnerable, oppressive, challenging, and passive – the impact of these ways of being need to be consistently considered and attended to through the workings of the relationship. I currently identify as a queer, African diasporan, able-bodied person. When working with a client who identifies as a queer, disabled, white English person, we may both experience oppression and privilege with each other differently at the location of the intersection of privilege, access, age, able-bodiedness, and nationality (ibid., p. 19). It is the work of intersectionality to collaboratively make meaning of these '*metaminorities*' (das Nair & Butler, 2012, p. 20) within the context of our therapeutic relationship, whilst considering how the dynamics promote or deny social justice.

Therapists, operating through intersectionality, often cultivate ways of working that foster 'antisubordination and social transformation' (May, 2015, p. 3). Therapy ought to be engaged with the political – what clients bring to the therapy room is not 'isolated personal phenomena, but as resulting from real life-conditions' (Glassgold & Drescher, 2011, p. 2). Suffering permeates life as a result of woundings from social relations and systems. Therapists are responsible for attending to how political realms impact clients (Avissar, 2016). To ignore conscious and unconscious suffering in the relationship is tantamount to social injustice. Being social justice-oriented, intersectionality in therapy must address systemic inequality by exposing ignorance, silence, and dominant oppressive structures. It is an act of social justice when clients voice oppression and privilege, transforming silence into the possibility of social change (Herman, 1997). It is an act of social justice when therapists actively engage with clients around these political matters. The more people are galvanised to affect personal change, the greater the potential for collective change that counteracts oppression (Glassgold, 2011).

The African Holocaust and enslavement legacies

The African Holocaust refers to the 'enslavement, colonisation, and oppression of African people' (Wong, 2016, p. 6). Alongside capitalism and the building of imperialism, some of the Holocaust's underpinning justifications were that Africans were seen as inferior to Europeans. It was deemed that in order for the souls of Africans to be saved, they needed to be converted to Christianity (ibid.) to receive their 'blessings' (Clarke, 1998). Many Africans lost the vast richness of their freedoms, intellectual capabilities, gender, sexuality and relationship customs, to become exploited and depicted as 'lesser being negroes'. Through a process of dehumanisation, the African Holocaust sought to destroy African peoples' memory, culture, customs, and documented history. The term 'enslavement' is used here, consciously and purposefully, to maintain the dignity of the African ancestors held in captivity, incriminating the inhumane responses of the white colonisers and their allies. The terms 'slave' and 'slavery' may be rendered outdated and inaccurate as they often omit a fuller context that 'enslavement' foregrounds and keeps conscious.

The transatlantic enslavement trade, also known as the middle passage, was part of the barbaric shipping system that captured Africans during the African Holocaust. Whilst empire and enslavement systems have long been part of human history – even within Africa itself – these were usually a result of war. Losers typically become indentured servitude, rather than chattel. What's pertinent about the African Holocaust is enslavement was based on 'racial inferiority' (DeGruy, 2005, p. 35) and provided the catalyst to turn business into an economy – building empires and funding large sections of the Global North.

DeGruy (2005) refers to 'Post Traumatic Slave Syndrome' as a condition that exists when a population has experienced multigenerational trauma resulting from centuries of enslavement, which manifests as continued oppression and systemic racism today. However, it seems more apt to refer to Post Traumatic '*Enslavement*' Syndrome', to consider queer African diasporan people's oppression and traumatisation at the intersection of ancestral lineage, class, wealth, educational access, sexuality, and gender. Such transgenerational and intergenerational experiences of oppression cultivate 'scars in the victims and victors alike, scars that embed themselves in our collective psyches and are passed down through generations, robbing us of our humanity' (ibid., p. iv). Racialised trauma 'lives in our bodies, our cells, and the expression of our genes' (Menakem, 2021, p. x). For some queer African diasporans, these traumas have generated profound dissociation, numbing, and forgetting. For others, there may be the persistent rage that exists at 'the violence, degradation, and humiliation visited upon us, our ancestors, and our children; anger at being relegated to the margins of society in which we live' (DeGruy, 2005, p. 115).

Part of what can be traumatic for queer African diasporan people is being in relation to 'white-body supremacy' (Menakem, 2021, p. xv) and its often-dominant expressions of heterosexism. The long history of enslavement, police brutality, and institutionalised racism, alongside covert experiences of microaggressions, underpins this. White body supremacy may be further contextualised through 'colonial object relations' (Lowe, 2008), where it is commonplace in African diasporan/white relationships for the white object, in its capacity to reduce a whole person to a part – skin – to attempt to, or actually, control, 'dominate or degrade the black object' (ibid., p. 22). Whether this is disguised or blatant, it exists in the individual and collective psyche. Therapists working with intersectionality, and queer African diasporan people, must attend to, and collaboratively make meaning of, somatic responses to work with this wounding, rather than rely on intellectualising (Menakem, 2021, p. 5) because trauma is held in the body. Therapists can support client's Sankofa quest through explorations of what it might mean to come home through the individual and collective body and its individual and collective wounds.

Sankofa: reclaiming eggs

Sankofa's quest and the cultivation of homecomings for African queer beings necessitates deconstructing imposed colonial and neo-colonial binary categorisations of how gender, sexuality, and relationship diversity are conceived. Sankofa's quest invites clients and therapists to look back and return with eggs/values/traditions that recognise how African people enjoyed myriad ways of being that existed before imperialistic, reductive, white racist conceptions. African-centred homecomings include reclaiming values that pre-date imperialism. Colonial conceptions have influenced decades of laws, policies, ostracisms, rapes, homicides, incarcerations, and death penalties (Matabeni & Pereira, 2014). Conversion practices and damning religious rhetoric that underpin cultural and familial values have spurred vitriol to condemn queer African diasporan people. Many African diasporan communities and their leaders have been vociferous in maintaining the colonial masters' own 'force, brutality, paternalism, arrogance, insensitivity and humiliation' (Tamale, 2011, p. 15). Often, the enslaved 'identify so closely with their tormentors that they become like them' (De Gruy, 2005, pp. 116–117). Heralding urgency, Sankofa – return (san), go (ko), take (fa) – signals the importance of redeeming African-centred ways of being.

Imperialists naively depicted African expressions of gender, sexuality, and relationships 'as primitive, exotic and bordering on nymphomania, but also it was perceived as immoral, bestial and lascivious. Africans were caricatured as having lustful dispositions' (Tamale, 2011, p. 15). Whilst lustfulness isn't inherently wrong, contextualising underpinning religious frameworks provides context for colonisers' wrongly conceived conceptions that undermined African ways of being. Colonial imposition of race as a categorisation tool, the violent split between ancestral lineage/legacy and sexuality, and the oppression experienced at this intersection, are part of the displacement that queer African diasporan people are affected by today. Thus, drawing on Sankofa's quest, there is a need for queer African diasporan clients to return home to gather the value of the eggs from a pre-colonial past, in order to consider the fullness of their decolonised, wholly African, erotic potential. The erotic, here, refers to a holistic sense of embodied freedom and aliveness.

With so much African-centred, undocumented and recounted history lost and denied, therapists concerned with the cultivation of homecomings must, as a means of psycho-education, be educated about African and world history to update and reframe clients' knowledge and their own potentially colonially-informed unconscious perspectives. There existed the 'Lovedu rain queen with her hundreds of wives . . . [and] . . . an early twentieth century female-husband among the Nuer in Sudan, Nandi in Kenya, Igbo in Nigeria or Fon in Dahomey (present-day Benin)' (Wieringa, 2005, pp. 281–282). There have been 'women marriages amongst the Kamba in Kenya and ancestral marriages of traditional healers (sangomas) in South Africa' (Morgan & Wieringa, 2005, p. 19). Yet, heterosexual sangomas now regard same-sex marriages as taboo. Present-day sangomas, who may be considered akin to younger lesbians, live openly in same-gender and non-binary relationships within urban contexts, yet older same-gender-identified sangomas maintain secrecy around their sexuality within traditional same-sex marriages (ibid.). It seems that where age intersects with gender and sexuality in these communities, privilege and oppression exist simultaneously. Whilst global influences impact upon ancient, localised customs, the sangomas suggest there are aspects of gender, sexuality, and relationship diversity that are wholly African and have been preserved. Further still, Dlamini (2006) highlights that the former leader of the Zulus, Shaka, insisted on a strict regime of same-gender relations for his warriors. Lewis (2011) offers a discussion about how a potential homoeroticism 'might have countenanced and even prescribed homosexuality for young men. Suggesting that homoeroticism among Zulu warriors was central to their definition of aggressive and triumphal masculinity' (p. 209). There is some danger in conflating historical ways of being queer, which relate back to the challenge of potentially interpreting African realities through European lenses. However, these examples offer scope to consider gender, relationship, and sexual diversity in pre-colonial societies that are not saturated by European imaginings or sensibilities.

Dlamini's (2006) research is particularly insightful to note how African sexuality 'was often defined in relation to reproduction, with the assumption being that Africans could not possibly display homoerotic desires or agencies, which were associated with sophisticated human desires and eroticism' (pp. 132–133). How sorrowful it is that African diasporan people maintain a legacy that is underpinned by colonial, patriarchal, racist assumptions that relate to economy and power, denying the rich legacies that the colonialists couldn't decipher. Epprecht's (2008) *Ethnography of African Straightness* noted how 'anthropologists "conscripted" select evidence and even fabricated "facts" about the people they studied in order to advance ideals and preferences concerning gender and sexuality in their own societies' (p. 34). It's a travesty that rights and liberties are still being denied on the basis of fabricated, outdated lies that are weaved through the collective psyche as though they were truths. When working with clients, therapists must interrogate these falsehoods in the cultivation of homecomings for queer African diasporan people. This deep-rooted psychological poison may be remedied as a means of social justice. Part of the remedy necessitates therapists facing 'the over-whelming and terrifying possibility that there are no models, that we shall have to create from scratch' (Bambara, 1970, p. 109). Starting from scratch signals a necessary and critical embodiment of Sankofa!

Nyumbani-Kuja

To explore what intersectionality *can do* in practice, consider Nyumbani-Kuja, a 23-year-old, queer-identified, Muslim, Tanzanian professional swimmer. Initially, they contacted me for therapy because they felt they were underperforming for their team; they'd lost their passion for the sport and felt suicidal. They wanted a confidential place to speak about microaggressions they were experiencing. Nyumbani-Kuja felt too weak to challenge the structure of the profession they felt privileged to be a part of, whilst feeling mute and invisible.

When working with clients, it can be helpful to have a working, flexible, inter-sectional hypothesis to support meaning-making. An intersectional hypothesis cultivates insight and exploration into the potential meaning that may be made of clients' presenting issues, suffering, and relationship to power structures. An inter-sectional hypothesis is to be held lightly, without certainty; it provides potential ways of seeing and gaining insight into the client's experience of 'social inequal-ity, intersecting power relations, social context, relationality, social justice, and complexity' (Collins & Bilge, 2020, p. 31).

I wondered about the emerging hypothesis of the unfolding story of a long-ing orphan. How would our therapeutic relationship reveal the wound within the heartache and the cry of this longing soul? I held an image of Nyumbani-Kuja's tiny being suffocated in a coffin, squashed by towering buildings. Rather than seek to resolve their suffering, I remained curious about these unconscious messages and the symbols offered that couldn't yet be articulated through coherent words. I was also curious about the absence of their sharing about home life and roots. I noticed embodied counter-transference: a hollow, empty feeling in my stom-ach; nervousness to speak. Nine months into our work, Nyumbani-Kuja shared a dream:

> Suffocated within a combusting railway train in Glasgow, Nyumbani-Kuja was trapped between two school buildings. Panicked, they vomited. The train descended into darkness. An emaciated, medal-wearing Christopher Columbus, offered faeces-filled water to drink. Columbus' brass-ringed fin-gers clenched a dagger and sliced off Nyumbani-Kuja's tongue. Screaming internally with familiar silent paralysis, Nyumbani-Kuja became mute. Water

gushed from Nyumbani-Kuja's mouth, ceasing the advancing flames. Suddenly, Nyumbani-Kuja's breastfeeding maternal Great-Grandmother and several unidentifiable rainbow-flag-wearing elders welcomed Nyumbani-Kuja into a palace. A coffin and cradle lay together in the middle of a pool. As Nyumbani-Kuja climbed veranda steps, their father, who resembled a small child, poured liquid into three golden chalices. The child beckoned Nyumbani-Kuja to drink. Clasping a dagger, the Great-Grandmother sliced Nyumbani-Kuja's hands, inviting them to choose whether to sleep in a coffin or cradle.

Nyumbani-Kuja wept through the retelling of their dream. Deeply moved, it felt important that I resist offering interpretations to give the dream and the powerful evoked feelings space, time, and attention. Over several months, we gently returned to this unconscious offering from the dream world. Amplifying their initial sense of being perplexed, they made meaning of how Glasgow benefitted from the enslavement trade – its initial railway network had received large sums of money from enslavement owners. Nyumbani-Kuja recognised Columbus as an overseeing, murdering figure of the African Holocaust – with blood on their hands, unduly heralded as a hero. They recognised how their own tongue felt silenced and saw the therapy as transforming the bloody wound to retrieve their own water of life. Nyumbani-Kuja saw the breastfeeding Grandmother figure and rainbow-flag-wearing elders as representative of the archetypal parents welcoming them home into a sexuality they were yet to fully embrace. They saw the small child as representing the innocence of a time before African fathers were ripped away from their children. They considered the gold as a chance to drink from their own forgotten stories – a necessary resourcing from deprivation and displacement and never feeling at home. They saw their cry for death, through suicide, as a longing to connect with home and parents they initially struggled to speak of. I remained curious about the amputation image and somatic tongue tingling.

As months went by, working with intersectionality seemed helpful to expose how oppressed and sad Nyumbani-Kuja felt in a swim team that ostracised them. Yet, the swim team were heralded as diversity champions. This echoed a quality of the Columbus character from the dream. Initially, Nyumbani-Kuja felt proud of their team's public image, and they benefited from capital gained from corporate sponsorship. Yet, beyond diversity posters that seemed focused on skin colour as explicit inclusion, Nyumbani-Kuja experienced a distinct lack of respect for their religious and cultural needs. Nyumbani-Kuja felt marginalised within a social context. Unlike their peers, Nyumbani-Kuja had won a scholarship to attend a prestigious school. They felt they had to remain silent about systemic racism, classism, queerphobia, and islamophobia to safeguard their precarious immigration status in the UK. They felt squashed between reverencing the tenets of their religion and fitting in with the swim team. When it emerged that they were dyslexic, they were taunted by coaches for making mistakes with paperwork. There seemed to be a pattern in their life of simultaneously being celebrated and privileged, alongside being oppressed and excluded, leaving them feeling subordinate and separate when in relationships.

Nyumbani-Kuja was often silent in therapy. Through embodied countertransference, I experienced a constricted throat, raised heartbeat, and sweaty palms. This seemed to express what they couldn't voice – feeling constricted by the 'structural, cultural, interpersonal power dynamics' with me and the swim team (ibid., p. 33). Nyumbani-Kuja feared the shame of not being believed by me, being depicted as 'having a chip on their shoulder', and becoming more ostracised and losing their corporate sponsorships. They feared losing what they had worked for and the identity they had gained in their local community as a success story. We attended to the power dynamics between us: my presenting characteristics as a queer African diasporan person made me safe enough to talk to, yet their East African family members had taught them not to trust 'dreadlocked Jamaicans', like me. They resented paying me and often paid late. We had to attend to this deep-seated prejudice and shadism. My complexion was lighter than theirs, and they considered themself ugly in my presence. I reminded them of their older sibling, who classified them as a weak liar. A negative transference often raged unrelentingly between us and had to be consistently negotiated and amplified to make meaning and address wounding. Intimacy between us was mediated by many moments of tender attunement, mutual non-defensive and authentic humour, playfulness, and a named sense of kinship that explicitly attended to the cultural pain, trauma, and power dynamics between us.

In the midst of one session, Nyumbani-Kuja described having an 'outer body experience' and could not attest to any real memory of cutting, swallowing pills, and contacting me from the hospital, following a suicide attempt. They barely recognised who they had become. They pleaded with me to know that 'this wasn't them'. Yet, the cutting experiences seemed to be a part of them that they couldn't make meaning of or accept. As our relationship deepened, Nyumbani-Kuja found the courage to say that a year prior to our meeting, their parents had been killed in a car collision. With just seven days of compassionate leave, they were expected to compete in tournaments when all they had known as 'home' seemed to disappear. The more they swam, the emptier they felt. They described a sense of feeling amputated, which they seemed to literalise symbolically through cutting. Returning to their dream, we hypothesised whether the hand slicing was symbolic of an initiation for one of their homecomings: returning to death – symbolised through the coffin – to cradle new ways of living. These fertile images seemed to reflect the transformative element of the retrieved Sankofa egg – found through looking back in order to look forward. Engagement with Sankofa's quest evoked their feelings of being mentally, physically, emotionally, and spiritually displaced. Divorced from structures that had once held them safe, they were paralysed within a wounded state. Wandering through a succession of one-night stands, they couldn't satisfy the abrupt loss of connection. They felt as though they belonged nowhere. They were separated from a sense of 'self' and all they had known, hence the incessant attempts to attach outwardly, rather than return home inwardly. They felt trapped in a coffin, a cycle of brokenness and separation, and couldn't fathom what reconnection could mean for them in reality. Multi-layered grief deepened the context for our work; it provided amplification for the image I held of feeling suffocated in a coffin – through the lightly-held, working intersectional hypothesis.

Exploring suicide with Nyumbani-Kuja revealed their desire to experience 'nothingness'. My task was not to panic and bypass their reality through an over-emphasis on ethical codes, which can so often reduce psychological thinking and negate the complexities of the context. My task was to bear with the psychological reality that Nyumbani-Kuja found untenable (Hillman, 2020, p. 22). There seemed to be a fantasy about entering 'nothingness' through death; our work deepened into exploring it. Nyumbani-Kuja wasn't expressing wishes to give up on life in its totality. They still had dreams, but they were lost. Their parents' deaths confronted them with a reality they couldn't shield from. Suicide seemed like a potential attempt to get into the heart of the phenomenon that was holding them hostage. Our relationship offered a bridge to enter the death experience that they were seeking to literalise (ibid., p. 71). It was necessary for us to enter the suicide fantasies so that Nyumbani-Kuja could experience death psychologically. Nyumbani-Kuja expressed their despair: some of this in relation to their parents, some of this transgenerational – much of this defended against. Space was made to lament their parents' deaths through rage and sorrow. Through Nyumbani-Kuja's grief, psychologically, we entered emptiness, which was part of the fantasy they thought the suicide would provide.

Thrice weekly sessions provided scope for Nyumbani-Kuja and I to deepen into their lived and ancestral reality and legacy of despair at homelessness. A keen Pan-Africanist, they were sorrowful about the rich legacy of African-centred history and discourse that they did not know about and wanted to reclaim as a pursuit of Sankofa. Yet, further cultivation of homecomings demanded that we gave a place to the utter awfulness of homelessness – as part of the diaspora; as being the only child of two parents who had died; of potentially losing their actual home if they did not fulfil the contractual obligations with the swim team. Our work was not to face into a home, in the first instance, but to face into the void of homelessness and absence – the very thing they wanted to transcend through suicide and death. The psychological task was not to revive hope. Our work was to do nothing but bear the agony of their parents' deaths and the soul's cry of the transgenerational trauma they experienced ancestrally. By simply being present in their experience of awfulness, there was space for Nyumbani-Kuja to do what they had never had the space to do: express themself as they were and have a voice. This was social justice in action: actively responding to the injustice of invisibility and voicelessness. Nyumbani-Kuja needed to know they weren't burdening me. It wasn't my responsibility to make things better. Doing so would have inadvertently left them alone, which is what they were already experiencing. The cultivation of homecomings with this queer African diasporan meant being with things as they were, rather than ridding myself of suffering prematurely. Integrating Sankofa's quest in the therapeutic work meant turning back with them to be in 'their death lands', 'the rage to live had passed' (ibid., p. 73), and we were not yet sure what was to be retrieved. Bearing with the agony, without resolve, is a necessary practice for therapists working with clients at these thresholds.

Nyumbani-Kuja began to understand their cutting as their cry for death; they didn't want help. Help would have robbed them of their death experience. The paradox was that by accepting their wish for death, the attempt at actually ending their life was abated, and they weren't so caught in the grip of having to transcend (ibid., p. 74). Social justice, through our work, meant that the oppression and grief that they were engulfed by had an opportunity to transform its initial weight. Practically, what intersectionality did for Nyumbani-Kuja was to bring them face to face with the complexities of grief, identity politics, power dynamics, the necessity of suicide and its ideation, and the power of cultivating homecomings through the therapeutic relationship. Questions of homecomings necessitate questions of homelessness and the distress that occurs without a place of belonging and home. When 'home' cannot be found wherever we might experience ourselves, death is often summoned for what feels unbearable to literalise part of the psyche's unfolding story.

Reclaiming de-colonised inheritances and erotic wholeness

Oftentimes, the quest for Sankofa cannot be sought without making space for lamentation and grief. Therapy attends to life as a whole; that work is continuous. As such, 'while it may be true that there are no real endings, no final homecomings . . . it is equally true that there are endings, homecomings, and destinations everywhere' (Eisenstein, 2017, p. xi). African-centred homecomings are referred to in their plurality as there are often many ongoing, cyclical processes of looking back, gathering, deepening; cultivating potential. For Nyumbani-Kuja, homecomings necessitated engaging with despair, rather than transcending it. Connecting with longings for death and re-birth, through their dream images of the coffin and cradle, through Sankofa's quest, Nyumbani-Kuja returned to face what had been lost and the gift and value in their lived and ancestral histories. By taking time to mourn, re-engaging with the nourishment of those attachments as a part of a cycle of homecomings, and returning to redeem their ancestral roots, Nyumbani-Kuja was no longer so trapped in cycles of lamentation for what they hoped for life to be. They began to attend to life as it was – this was central to many of their continual homecomings. For some clients, it may seem impossible to find 'home', despite being haunted by its relentless longing and mysterious allure of reconciliation (Akomolafe, 2017b). Still, therapy may act as a container to attend to Sankofa's quest – grieving what has been dislocated (ibid., p. 154), alongside reclaiming fragments, that must be ingested, in the return to one's inheritance, wisdom, and customs. Clients, like Nyumbani-Kuja, may build shrines as outward symbols that cultivate internalised homecomings, honouring loss, re-membering, deepening connection, and belonging.

When cultivating queer African diasporan homecomings and therapy with clients, therapists are invited to become agents for systemic change, who traverse the 'intersection between therapist/activist identities' (das Nair & Butler, 2012, p. 5). Therapists must re-educate themselves about how gender, sexuality, and relationship diversity might be deconstructed to release colonial baggage. In terms of Sankofa's quest, whilst aspects of African-centred history and discourse are denied and forgotten, perhaps this chapter can galvanise action and support therapists who work with queer African diasporan clients. Clients may be supported in their conscious and unconscious longings and expressed needs to reclaim their decolonised inheritance and erotic wholeness by embodying the freedom to consider what being at home in themselves might mean to them. Therapists are invited to integrate African-centred perspectives, such as Sankofa and its quest, into their practice and to re-think the origins and implications of imperialistic theories and practices that dominate and subordinate their clients and themselves.

Though anchors and references for home may sometimes feel troublesome to source for queer African diasporan people, like myself, the writing of this chapter has provided opportunities to engage with my own quest of Sankofa. Taking hold of the symbolic dagger from Nyumbani-Kuja's dream, deconstructing colonised and decolonised re-education, psychotherapeutic discourse and therapeutic approaches, buries the coffins. In turn, we may cultivate re-visioned realms for fertile cradles where we, as therapists, through the capacity of wounded healing, alongside queer African diasporan clients, can continue in the process of recovering from the imposition of colonial muzzles and shackles that have permeated the psyche. Accordingly, we can actively and consciously engage with the freedom, right, and necessity of keeping our heads looking back, returning, gathering, reclaiming, with forward-facing feet, owning and stepping into the fullness of our own queer, erotic potential. Sankofa!

References

Akomolafe, A. C. (2017a). Beyond truth: The subversion of story. In A. C. Akomolafe, M. K. Asante, & A. Nwoye (Eds.), *We Will Tell Our Own Story, The Lions of Africa Speak!* New York: Universal Write Publications LLC.

Akomolafe, B. (2017b). *These Wilds Beyond Our Fences, Letters to My Daughter on Humanity's Search for Home*. Berkely, CA: North Atlantic Books.

Allen, J. S. (2012). Black/queer/diaspora at the current conjuncture. *GLQ, A Journal of Lesbian and Gay Studies, 18*(2–3). Duke University Press.

Avissar, N. (2016). *Psychotherapy, Society, and Politics, From Theory to Practice*. New York: Palgrave Macmillan.

Bailey, A. (2010). On intersectionality and the whiteness of feminist philosophy. In G. Yancy (Ed.), *The Center Must Not Hold: White Women Philosophers on the Whiteness of Philosophy*. Lanham, MD: Lexington Books.

Bambara, T. C. (1970). On the issue of roles. In *The Black Woman: An Anthology*. New York: Mentor.

Belkin, M. (2020). Who is queer around here? In M. Belkin & C. White (Eds.), *Intersectionality and Relational Psychoanalysis*. London and New York: Routledge.

Cho, S., Crenshaw, K. W., & McCall, L. (2013). Toward a field of intersectionality studies: Theory, applications, and praxis. *Signs, 38*(4), 785–810.

Clarke, J. H. (1998). *Christopher Columbus and the Afrikan Holocaust, Slavery and the Rise of European Capitalism*. Buffalo, NY: Eworld Inc.

Cohen, C. J. (2005). Punks, bulldaggers, and welfare queens: The radical potential of queer politics? In E. P. Johnson & M. G. Henderson (Eds.), *Black Queer Studies: A Critical Anthology*. Durham and London: Duke University Press.

Collins, P. H. (2000). *Black Feminist Thought: Knowledge, Consciousness, and the Politics of Empowerment* (2nd ed.). New York: Routledge.

Collins, P. H., & Bilge, S. (2020). *Intersectionality*. Cambridge and Medford, MA: Polity Press.

Crenshaw, K. W. (2011). Postscript. In H. Lutz, M. T. H. Vivar, & L. Supik (Eds.), *Framing Intersectionality: Debates on a Multi-Faceted Concept in Gender Studies*. Farnham: Ashgate.

das Nair, R., & Butler, C. (2012). *Intersectionality, Sexuality and Psychological Therapies: Working with Lesbian, Gay and Bisexual Diversity*. Chichester, West Sussex: BPS Blackwell and John Wiley and Sons Ltd.

DeGruy, J. (2005). *Post Traumatic Slave Syndrome: America's Legacy of Enduring Injury and Healing*. Portland, OR: Joy DeGruy Publications Inc.

Diop, C. A. (1991). *Civilization or Barbarism: An Authentic Anthropology* Salemson, H. J., de Jager, M., trans., & Yaa-Lengi, M. N., eds.). Chicago: Lawrence Hill Books. Originally published as *Civilisation ou Barbarie: Anthropologie Sans Complisance (1981)*. Paris: Présence Africaine.

Dlamini, B. (2006). Homosexuality in the African context. *Agenda, 67*, 128–136.

Eisenstein, C. (2017). Foreword. In B. Akomolafe (Ed.), *These Wilds Beyond Our Fences, Letters to My Daughter on Humanity's Search for Home*. Berkely, CA: North Atlantic Books.

Epprecht, M. (2008). *Heterosexual Africa? The History of an Idea from the Age of Exploration to the Age of Aids*. Pietermariztburg, South Africa: University of KwaZulu-Natal Press.

Glassgold, J. M. (2011). *Dreams Begin Responsibilities Psychology, Agency, and Activism* in *Activism in LGBT Psychotherapy Practice*. New York: Haworth Medical Press.

Glassgold, J. M., & Drescher, J. (Eds.). (2011). *Activism in LGBT Psychotherapy Practice*. New York: Haworth Medical Press.

Herman, J. A. (1997). *Trauma and Recovery: The Aftermath of Violence-from Domestic to Violence to Political Terror*. New York: Basic Books.

Hillman, J. (2020). *Suicide and the Soul*. New York: Spring Publications.

Johnson, E. P. (2005). "Quare" studies, or (almost) everything I know about queer studies I learned from my grandmother. In E. P. Johnson & M. G. Henderson (Eds.), *Black Queer Studies: A Critical Anthology*. Durham and London: Duke University Press.

Johnson, E. P., & Henderson, M. G. (2005). *Black Queer Studies: A Critical Anthology*. Durham and London: Duke University Press.

Lewis, D. (2011). Representing African sexualities. In S. Tamale (Eds.), *African Sexualities, A Reader*. Fahamu, Dakar, Nairobi, and Oxford: Pambazuka Press.

Lowe, F. (2008). Colonial object relations: Going underground Black and White relations. *British Journal of Psychotherapt, 24*(1), 20–33. Oxford and Malden, MA, BAP and Blackwell Publishing Ltd.

Matebeni, Z., & Pereira, J. (2014). Preface. In E. F. White (Ed.), *Reclaiming Afrikan, Queer Perspectives on Sexual and Gender Identities*. Athlone, South Africa: Modaji Books.

May, V. M. (2015). *Pursuing Intersectionality: Unsettling Dominant Imaginaries*. New York and London: Routledge.

Mazama, A. (2017). Afrocentricity and the critical question of African agency. In A. C. Akomolafe, M. K. Asante, & A. Nwoye (Eds.), *We Will Tell Our Own Story, The Lions of Africa Speak*! New York, Universal Write Publications LLC.

Menakem, R. (2021). *My Grandmother's Hands: Racialized Trauma and the Pathway to Mending Our Hearts and Bodies*. London: Penguin Books.

Morgan, R., & Wieringa, S. (2005). *Tommy Boys, Lesbian Men and Ancestral Wives: Female Same-Sex Practices in Africa*. Johannesburg, South Africa: Jacana Media (Pty) Ltd.

Muñoz, J. B. (2009). *Cruising Utopia, the Then and There of Queer Futurity*. New York and London: New York University Press.

Nyanzi, S. (2014). Queering Queer Africa. In E. F. White (Ed.), *Reclaiming Afrikan, Queer Perspectives on Sexual and Gender Identities*. Athlone, South Africa: Modaji Books.

Romero, M. (2018). *Introducing Intersectionality*. Cambridge and Medford, MA: Polity Press.

Tamale, S. (2011). *African Sexualities, A Reader*. Fahamu, Dakar, Nairobi, and Oxford: Pambazuka Press.

Wieringa, S. (2005). Chapter nine. In R. Morgan & S. Wieringa (Eds.), *Tommy Boys, Lesbian Men and Ancestral Wives: Female Same-Sex Practices in Africa*. Johannesburg, South Africa: Jacana Media (Pty) Ltd.

Willis, W. B. (1998). *The Adinkra Dictionary, A Visual Primer on the Language of Adinkra*. Washington, DC: Pyramid Complex.

Wong (Omowale), D. (2016). *The Devastation and Economics of the African Holocaust*. Scotts Valley, CA: CreateSpace Independent Publishing Platform.

Chapter 8

Working with intimate partner violence in **GSRD** intimate relationships

Rima Hawkins

Intimate partner violence (IPV) is probably as common in GSRD communities as it is in heterosexual cisgendered monogamous relationships. I will address the issues relating to domestic abuse in intimate relationships in the GSRD community that therapists need to be aware of and help them recognise the signs and symptoms in their therapy space.

Safety first

Before we start, let's position ourselves in safety. Given the high prevalence of abuse and violence in our society, I am aware that therapists themselves may have faced such experiences, and this chapter may be a difficult read. This triggering potential might be further increased if you are part of the marginalised communities that this chapter considers. I urge you to take good care of yourself whilst reading. Take breaks, read another chapter, employ your self care strategies as and when you need to. This is a good model to use in therapy sessions where such breaks with clients can be helpful.

This chapter addresses the basics a therapist needs to know about the law with regard to intimate partner violence (IPV), rather than detailing the comprehensive legal framework pertaining to it. There are resources and links listed at the end of the chapter should you wish to explore the law more in depth. In the UK, laws are implemented differently in each of the jurisdictions: Scotland, Wales, Northern Ireland and England. For the purposes of this chapter all legal discussions are based on the legal proceedings of England and Wales. Scotland, Northern Ireland and other parts of the world will have their own legal framework with regards to IPV and sexual violence (SV). If you are working with a case of abuse and/ or violence outside England and Wales, please check the laws in your client's jurisdiction.

When clients present with IPV, you will need to assess if you can work with them or need to make a referral to a specialist service for therapy. This chapter enables you to understand the issues related to IPV which may require specialist input. If you want to work with IPV with any client group, you will need

DOI: 10.4324/9781003260561-9

to undertake specific trainings that cover the legal dimension, pre-trial therapy requirements, safeguarding, safety planning, trauma and shame work. Specialist supervision is also recommended.

Language and terminology

In this chapter, I have used GSRD/LGBTQIA+ communities interchangeably based on the context. Domestic abuse and sexual violence within intimate relationships are also defined as IPV, and this is used interchangeably. Language and terminology in this field is sensitive and loaded in addition to the sensitivities of the GSRD world. The word 'abuse' has connotations of manipulation or exploitation over a period of time, whereas the word 'violence' has nuances of fierceness, ferocity and viciousness associated with it. In my experience, both abuse and violence, however deployed, can have psychological and physical impacts on a person. There are legal frameworks which clarify and define these behaviours in legal terminology; however, we also develop our own lines and boundaries within which we accept certain behaviours influenced by many factors, such as culture and politics. It is crossing that personal line that makes a client want to seek help to further explore meaning of their experiences and choices they have.

When people experience abuse or violence, they are called 'victims of crime', 'survivors' or, if they have reported the crime to the criminal justice system, they are called 'complainants'. The abuser is called the 'perpetrator', 'persecutor' or 'offender' and, in the criminal justice system, they are called the 'defendant' or the 'suspect'. It is important to note that sometimes in relationships both partners can be victims and offenders. It is important to ask the client what terminology they would be comfortable with, if referred to about them.

Clients choose words to reflect their subjective process to make sense of the event and what happened to them. Their choice of words might be different to legal or professional language. As with most instances in therapy, we can ask a client which words they would prefer to use and, when the time is right, unpack the meanings behind those words for the client. However, in the GSRD community, clients' pronouns need to be respected rather than explored.

Definitions

It may be useful to understand the differences between interpersonal violence and intimate partner violence and how IPV in both contexts is defined internationally and nationally. The Violence Prevention Alliance (VPA) is a network of the World Health Organisation (WHO) Member States, international agencies and civil society organizations working to prevent violence. VPA participants share an evidence-based public health approach that targets the risk factors leading to violence and promotes multi-sectoral cooperation. Participants are committed to implementing the recommendations of the World Report on Violence and Health. The VPA defines **violence** as:

> the intentional use of physical force or power, threatened or actual, against oneself, another person, or against a group or community, that either results in or has a high likelihood of resulting in injury, death, psychological harm, maldevelopment, or deprivation.
>
> (www.who.int/violenceprevention/en/)

VPA's definition includes interpersonal violence in their general definition of violence. Interpersonal violence refers to violence between individuals and is subdivided into family and intimate partner violence and community violence. The former category includes child maltreatment, intimate partner violence and elder abuse, while the latter is broken down into acquaintance and stranger violence and includes youth violence, assault by strangers, violence related to property crimes and violence in workplaces and other institutions.

Collective violence refers to violence committed by larger groups of individuals and can be subdivided into social, political and economic violence. Honour based crimes and female genital mutilation (FGM) form part of this definition.

Previously, sexual violence was seen to be separate to domestic violence, but following research, it was established that sexual violence is more likely to occur within intimate relationship than strangers (Campbell & Soeken, 1999). Sexual violence, therefore, was included in the Domestic Abuse definition and together referred to as IPV. The World Health Organization (2012) defines **sexual violence** as:

> any sexual act, attempt to obtain a sexual act, unwanted sexual comments or advances, or acts to traffic, or otherwise directed, against a person's sexuality using coercion, by any person regardless of their relationship to the victim, in any setting, including but not limited to home and work.

In the UK, the legal age to consent to have sex is 16 years irrespective of sexuality or gender. Under the Sexual Offences Act 2003, people under the age of 13 years cannot give consent. There are other issues such as capacity and freedom to consent to be considered whilst considering consent.

The UK cross government definition of **domestic violence and abuse** is covered in the legal frameworks of the Domestic abuse Act 2021 and Sexual Offences Act 2003:

> any incident or pattern of incidents of controlling, coercive, threatening behaviour, violence or abuse between those aged 16 or over who are, or have been, intimate partners or family members regardless of gender or sexuality.

The abuse can encompass, but is not limited to: psychological, physical, sexual, financial, emotional.

(Home Office, 2013)

Domestic abuse (also called intimate partner violence) can include, but is not limited to, the following:

- Coercive control (a pattern of intimidation, degradation, isolation and control with the use or threat of physical or sexual violence).
- Verbal abuse or vilification.
- Psychological and/or emotional abuse.
- Physical or sexual abuse.
- Financial or economic abuse.
- Online or digital abuse.
- Stalking and harassment.
- Family violence such as forced marriage, female genital mutilation and so called 'honour crimes'.

Prevalence

Public stories construct domestic violence as a gendered, heterosexual phenomenon that is predominantly physical in nature (Donovan & Hester, 2010). Most studies in the areas of IPV, however, find prevalence rates among LGBTQ people to be as high as or higher than those of the general population or in heterosexual groups (Donovan & Hester, 2010). The Crime Survey for England and Wales (CSEW), for the year ending March 2020, showed that an estimated 2.3 million adults aged 16 to 74 years experienced domestic abuse in the last year. This equates to a prevalence rate of approximately 5 in 100 adults (5%). In contrast, research conducted by Stonewall (2018) shows that more than "one in ten LGBT people (11 per cent) have faced domestic abuse from a partner in the last year. This increases to 17 per cent of Black, Asian and minority ethnic LGBTQ people". IPV rates in same-sex relationships range from 25% to 50% (Carvalho et al., 2011), and between 31% and 50% of trans people experience IPV over their lifetime (Brown & Herman, 2015).

According to most literature available based on prevalence, it is believed that IPV is gender-based violence, deeply rooted in the societal inequality between men and women. More recently, there has been acknowledgement that men and minority groups like LGBTQ folk are victims of IPV, but the characteristics of these groups are often not acknowledged for many reasons and therefore the difference in the impact is little understood (Davies & Neal, 1996). If it was true that violence is only gender based, then female same-sex partners in an intimate relationship would be less likely to experience abuse and violence compared to male same-sex partners. According to Stonewall (2018), 13% of bi women and 10% of lesbians have experienced IPV in a relationship, with a woman being the perpetrator in two-thirds of these cases. There is limited research on trans people. One study directly compared the lifetime prevalence of IPV among transgender and cisgender people and found that 31.1% of transgender people and 20.4% of cisgender people had ever experienced IPV or dating violence (Langenderfer-Magruder et al., 2016). We know that reporting of crime is a complex issue, and many victims don't report or disclose, so the data we have is likely to be the tip of the iceberg.

Studies by Karakurt et al. (2021) show a range of 40% to 91% of women experiencing IPV have incurred a traumatic brain injury (TBI) due to physical assault (Campbell et al., 2018). More than two-thirds of IPV victims are strangled at least once – the average is 5.3 times per victim (Chrisler & Ferguson, 2006; Abbott et al., 1995; Coker et al., 2002). Strangulation was added to the list in the Domestic Abuse Act 2021 as part of the definition. It is a common form of physical violence, and even if it is not painful, it is still cutting off oxygen to the brain and can leave marks, make voice raspy, or break blood vessels in eyes. Victims can die from TBI hours or days after the assault.

Presentations of domestic abuse and sexual abuse can be different. The most common type of abuse experienced by GSRD people is verbal abuse, which is intended to offend, humiliate, intimidate, demean or frighten someone (e.g. abuse and harassment), rather than physical acts (e.g. violence) or sexual violence.

The data from Galop publications (Hubbard, 2021) concurs with the prevalence of verbal abuse (92%), followed by online abuse (60%) and harassment (59%). Physical violence was 29% and 17% was sexual violence. The number who were outed and doxed (posting private information of someone else online with malicious intent), which is a type of violence very specific to the GSRD community, was 28%. This research suggests that homophobia, biphobia, transphobia, acephobia and intersexphobia remain a substantial part of the lives of GSRD people, which can have significant consequences for those targeted. Due to the difficulty to access services for the support needed, many GSRD individuals continue to live with abuse and violence and normalise it as a defence or coping mechanism.

IPV in LGBTQIA+ intimate relationships

LGBTQIA+ hate crime is disproportionately on the rise in the UK. When minority groups experience hate crime, they often internalise this oppression, leading to minority stress, which leads to interpersonal prejudice and discrimination (Meyer et al., 2007).

The experience of abuse in GSRD communities is different in that victims can often experience abuse that is targeted at their gender identity and/or sexual orientation (Iantaffi, 2021). This can include actual or threatened outing of gender identity or sexual orientation to family, friends or in the workplace; being ridiculed for their gender identity or sexual orientation; having their identity denied and having their HIV status used against them. This vulnerability leads to the decreased reporting, abuse and violence repeating and forming patterns which are normalised. Experiences of discrimination from criminal justice or support professionals in the past has led to people in GSRD communities not seeking or finding help. It is important to know that there is no time limit for reporting to the police in the UK justice system. This gives time for the victim to think about whether or not they want to report or need time to feel psychologically and physically ready to be able to cope with the consequences of reporting.

Relationships fundamentally seek needs to be met by the other. Partners have to work at it, couples or polycules or polyamory, no matter how hard it gets and how much they change over time. As Meg-John Barker concludes, love hurts, but the choice people make is to stay together or move away seeking for the better suited relationship (see Barker & Gabb, 2016).

There are consequences of an unhappy relationship. They may start with unbearable conflicts moving and escalating to non-consensual dynamics such as violent behaviours which leads to a sense of deflation and failure (leading to shame and guilt). Violent behaviour can sometimes feel the only way to express the intensity of emotions such as frustration. Aggressive behaviour is not a linear movement of escalation but can happen at any stage in the relationship and in various forms, as defined previously, in any close intimate relationship. Clients continue to stay in a relationship for various reasons. The risk of leaving and risk of staying needs exploring.

Practices of love can be confused with practices of violence (I am hitting you or controlling your finances for your own good). This is a well-known phenomenon called 'trauma bond' (Jülich, 2005). It occurs when the abused person forms an unhealthy bond with the person who abuses them. The person experiencing abuse may develop sympathy for the abusive person, which becomes reinforced by cycles of abuse, followed by remorse. Lauren Kozlowski (2020) in her book *Trauma Bonding* explains stages that lead to becoming trauma bonded and the recovery journey.

This is one of the many reasons why partners stay in an abusive relationship and victims do not recognise their experience as abuse until much later in life. Behaviours include sexual practices too.

Consensual BDSM has become more mainstream but remains marginalised and misunderstood (Thompson, 2021). Understanding the culture of Kink and practices of BDSM that is consensual and intimacy-enhancing, and distinguishing it from non-consensual behaviours or harming (abuse) by way of this practice, is important. Therapists need not make an issue when there is none, nor pathologise or make assumptions about the practices of kink and BDSM but have the understanding to make appropriate assessment and intervention when there is an issue to be addressed (Shahbaz and Chirinos, 2017).

Impact of IPV in specific GSRD groups

It is common knowledge that victims of childhood sexual abuse are less likely to identify and express their relational needs as adults. As a result of low self-esteem, they may be an easy target for abuse such as IPV. The impacts and consequences experience include physical injuries, emotional and psychological impacts, financial costs and behaviour changes.

When clients experience IPV, it can destroy the trust and intimacy the relationship was built on. It is important to make an assessment and identify if the client is in crisis or dealing with trauma. Either way stabilisation of the client is important so that they are able to make the right decision for themselves. These may include grounding techniques, breathing exercises and slowing down the process.

Lesbians, bisexual women, heterosexual trans women

The definition of rape under the SO Act 2003 is penetration by a penis without consent. There is a gendered perception of members of the GSRD community identifying as women who experience sexual violence. Lesbians and bisexual women in same-sex relationships may be dismissed (Penone & Guarnaccia, 2018). Although bisexual women are 1.8 times more likely to report ever having experienced IPV than heterosexual women (Taylor & Herman, 2015). Trans women who have a penis may not be perceived as victims and be disregarded. It is important to encourage the ability to voice their expressions of their sexuality and gender identity even if the act of sexual violence may challenge this. The therapy space is a place where they can reclaim their own identity, including their sexuality and gender, which is crucial and healing and creates resilience in dealing with the trauma.

Gay, bisexual men, and trans men

The myth of masculinity is that men are not weak – they are not victims but are perpetrators. Men may question their experiences of violence and abuse as something shameful. The history of the gay movement challenged judgement and prejudices, and the community's memory of discriminations, assault, physical and psychological hurt is not easily forgotten. For gay and bisexual men, their internalised homophobia may create shame and self-blame in being in a same-sex relationship ('if I was in a heterosexual relationship, this would not happen to me'). The sense of deserved abuse and violence as a boy or an adult male silences them. More recently, those who experienced violence when engaged in chemsex may also fear moral judgements and worry they might get in trouble because of illegal drug use. They may also fear they would be outed as a result (Cavacuiti & Chan, 2008). The shame of trans men can be more intense as they may be in between gender bias of what it means to be a victim based on their perceived gender. In addition, if they had been sexually abused, their gender transitioning could be pathologised and perceived as their defence. Research from the Coral Project and Stonewall shows that more than a quarter of trans people (28%) in a relationship have faced domestic abuse from a partner.

Asexual people

There is a propensity to pathologise people who identify as asexual, believing that it is as a result of sexual abuse, or they just haven't found the right person to have sex with. They are infantalised as sexually immature. In my experience, they are also victims of the common confusion between gender and sexuality as people believe that those who transition do not have a sexuality because they are not within their binary belief (the same confusion happens in transitioning folks who are assumed to be changing their sexuality). It is common for asexual people to be victims of sexual abuse through compulsory sexuality beliefs (e.g. spouse threatening separation if the partner doesn't want or have sex). Moreover, because asexuality is defined as an absence of sexual desire, it is incorrectly assumed that they are not in intimate relationships and therefore invisible as victims of IPV.

Carmen Maria Machado (2020), in her book *In The Dream House* explores domestic abuse; the essay titled 'Dream House as Queer Villany' unpicks the 'problem and pleasure' of queer villains. In particular, Machado exposes the representational bind that LGBTQIA+ characters are disproportionately being forced to play the villain. Machado urges to keep the queer villains coming, but to place them alongside a diverse range of LGBTQIA+ characters, rather than include them in isolation. Narrated through the dual lens of past victim and then survivor of domestic abuse, the memoir makes an intervention into the gendered assumptions which overpower the conversations around abuse, by showing how it can develop between two women and how the shame of relationship failure keeps the abuse alive.

The SafeLives Report (2018) shows that victims of domestic abuse who identify as LGBTQIA+ are almost twice as likely to have attempted to take their own life, twice as likely to have self-harmed and more likely to experience mental health problems, highlighting the urgent need for specialist support and attention to the needs of LGBTQIA+ victims of IPV.

Cultural factors in GSRD people and IPV

Not all cultures adopt or are open to gender equality, and therefore some domestic abuse may be normalised, such as controlling women with their clothing, their activities and whom they choose to spend time with. In some cultures women's consent to have sex is not acknowledged. For people within those cultures, such behaviours may not be deemed as domestic abuse. There are some cultures where being GSRD is against the law with serious consequences. Some GSRD folks remain in heterosexual relationships, enduring abuse which is compounded trauma with repressing sexuality and being victims of IPV. Even if an individual is willing to disclose IPV, they may not be willing to say their partner is of the same-sex, and so any research or interventions may not accurately fit their situation due to the previously mentioned challenges unique to GSRD individuals (Baker et al., 2012).

The UK is liberal enough for GSRD communities to exist, but some people live within their original family and community cultural beliefs and values whereby there is a fear of speaking up about abuse. Socialised concepts of power dynamics, gender bias and what is considered 'normal' within sexuality vary from culture to culture.

This chapter cannot ignore the oppressions and abuse on GSRD people by the heteronormative culture. Some therapists who support the unethical corrective or conversion practices may promote that being in a same-sex relationship is abnormal and inherently abusive, colluding with the erasure of IPV within GSRD community. The lived experience of GSRD people of sexual abuse and/or violence and the choices people make when considering whether to speak up or keep quiet depends on how understood they feel. The fear is about the intrusiveness of questioning, expression of disbelief, disgust, or judgement, and for this they feel forced to explain their identities, language and community norms or risk a homophobic, biphobic or transphobic reaction from the person they tell.

Client presentations in therapy

As sex and relationship therapists (SRT), we are more likely to have clients with intimate partner violence (IPV) whether it be domestic or sexual. This is also because GSRD clients are less likely to have confidence in the police and the perceived incompetencies of the Criminal Justice System. Moreover, a client may be in denial or in trauma bond and not see abuse and violence as breaking boundaries but just as a reaction from the partner for what they have done wrong.

The GSRD community facing violence and abuse may not wish to report, due to well-established reasons of minority stress, internalised oppression and shame, and a history of homophobic and transphobic treatment. They fear being misunderstood, blamed, shamed and victimised.

Clients generally present in five categories for therapy.

A Carefully cognisant of the fact that they are starting to experience IPV and clients want help to stop the pattern and willing to change.
B They appear unhappy and depressed in their relationship and want to explore the reason for their unhappiness but without understanding the existence of IPV within the relationship.
C They are in a toxic abusive relationship where both or all intimate partners are in a pattern of abuse and stuck in the cycle of abuse or sexual violence which they find recurring but unable to change. There is presence of physical and/or emotional damage.
D Clients disclose a recent physical or sexual assault that may need forensics and legal documentation as evidence for court should the client decide to press charges at a later date.
E Client has already reported the abuse/violence and is waiting for the criminal justice system to take their case forward.

A and B are the two most common presentations in therapy. It is important to recognise through enquiry how easy or difficult accessing therapy has been for them. Whilst a therapist would explore with a client what their risks were, what makes them unhappy and if they are safe, there may also be an important issue of D as recent disclosure would need to be addressed. In some circumstances where the abuse is current and severe, clients have an option to disclose to the police and have rights to justice. This must be explored and not taken for granted. Any disclosure should follow documentation rules required by the Crown Prosecution Service (CPS).

Therapists must be knowledgeable and trained in pre-trial therapy (PTT) guidance issued by the CPS (2022) should they be working with the C and D category of clients. If they are not trained, they should make a referral to a specialist agency working with IPV.

If a client experienced sexual violence (rape or sexual assault) within the last seven days, they may still have the opportunity of giving forensic samples to a Sexual Assault Referral Centre (SARC) without reporting it to the police. This self-referral option gives clients and victims of sexual crime some time to think if they wish to report or not. The samples are kept anonymously for two years. There is also an option for the SARC to process the samples and identify if the offender has had previous convictions or similar cases reported. This can strengthen the case and encourage the client to report formally to get justice. Clients need to be given the opportunity and explained to them the benefit of doing this. Every county in England and Wales has a SARC associated with the police force. Therapists can find their local SARC details on search engines. Someone who has experienced physical violence should be referred to A&E for a physical check-up.

Appropriate interventions

For IPV the best risk assessment form to use is the Safelives risk checklist, which you can get from their website (safelives.org.uk).

The key model to use for IPV is a person-centred approach with a trauma informed lens, which includes the following:

- Safety.
- Trustworthiness and transparency.
- Peer support.
- Collaboration and mutuality.
- Empowerment, voice and choice.
- Cultural, historical, and gender issues.

Interventions to address IPV in GSRD relationships would be beneficial if the therapist's work included psychoeducation about dynamics of power and control within relationships and how the cycle of violence specifically affects the client work both on the individual and systemic levels. This can be done with the explanation of a power and control wheel, such as the one from the Domestic Abuse Intervention Project, provided by Duluth (theduluthmodel.org/wheels/).

Additionally, the therapist could provide GSRD-friendly community resources available for the client, such as local support groups. It would be also useful to warn clients of the shelters/refuge being heteronormative and potentially having very little understanding of GSRD issues.

Finally, the therapist could guide the client in safety planning. This process can include identifying people the client can reach out to for support and/or routes to get out of their home during an altercation. Safety planning and risk assessment should be conducted within each session as an ongoing process (SaveLives Report, 2018).

Information about safety plans and how to create them can be found on the following websites:

> Women's Aid (womensaid.org.uk)
> IDAS (idas.org.uk)
> My Sisters Place (mysistersplace.org.uk)

Case study

Shaun is an Irish, bisexual, cisgender man. He is 30 years old. He grew up in Ireland with strict Catholic upbringing. He has a close knit family of five brothers and ageing parents. All his brothers are married. As the youngest, he is the favourite of his parents, and they are keen he gets married soon. They know he is in a relationship. Shaun is seeing Cara who is trans femme (pronouns she/her). Cara was not introduced to Shaun's family. Shaun and Cara have a volatile relationship, often physical, when arguing followed by make-up sex. Cara is aware Shaun's parents are putting pressure on him to get married, and Shaun and Cara have agreed that they cannot be seen together in public or be married to protect Shaun from being ostracised by his family. Cara has threatened Shaun that if he leaves her, she will tell his family and expose their relationship and disclose her gender identity. Shaun has come for individual therapy seeking help as he 'feels trapped' and feels distressed as he is 'blackmailed by Cara'.

In the assessment session, I asked Shaun about the physical assaults and the impact it's had on him. Initially, he ignored the discussion about physical hitting, saying "this is part of the relationship, this is what we do". In further sessions, when we further discussed the emotional blackmail as identified by him, he began to talk about shame, isolation and feeling very cornered. He began to discuss power dynamics in the relationship and saw a pattern of abuse. He said that Cara doesn't recognise her controlling behaviour. We explored his tendency to appease Cara so he is able to have the relationship he wants, but at the same time he is aware he has to accept violence and emotional abuse to get what he wants. The exploration also involved how he learnt to appease his family of origin, concealing his sexuality to maintain status quo culturally.

Shaun's own threshold for bearing physical pain is high, and he has developed his owns lines or boundaries for tolerating it by make-up sex. This experience of trauma and joy or cruelty and kindness bound together creates a belief that pain will not last long, and the pleasure following pain can be very gratifying. In my experience with clients, some GSRD individuals will bear emotional abuse longer than others due to internalised oppression, whereas the same individuals may have a low threshold for physical abuse because they are used to protecting themselves in physical spaces. I think this is because physical abuse is an action defined by visible impact such as bruises. Emotional coercion or other types of abuse may be subtle and may become invisible within a daily relationship.

Assessment

Following a general assessment, I asked Shaun the following questions:

- Are you safe, or is your life at risk?

  He said his life wasn't at risk, but he risked losing his family. His sexuality would be outed. There were other implications.

- Do you want to (a) leave or (b) stay in this relationship?

  He wanted to stay in this relationship. I explored with him the consequences of staying and what he wanted to change to make him feel safe and how he could be in this relationship.

  If he had said he wanted to leave the relationship, I would have asked him what were the implications and how could he mitigate them safely:

  - Are you safe to leave your partner?
  - Are you ready to leave the relationship?

Risk assessment is the first step towards ensuring the client's safeguarding needs. This would entail the client reporting to authorities for his own safety. Therapists working in an organisation may need to disclose if the client's life or any children may be in danger. If the therapist is a private practitioner, they do not have any responsibility to disclose IPV.

Shaun's assessment showed coercive control and physical abuse by definition of the law, I made a mental note of it but did not say this to Shaun. Shaun felt 'trapped' and 'blackmailed'. These were Shaun's words. This is important because if this case went to court and I, as the therapist, identified the definition of what was going on, it could be deemed as coaching the victim, and the case may be dismissed on those grounds only. The client has to describe the events in their own words. Therapists should take factual notes of the events just in case their notes are subpoenaed.

When clients come to see a therapist with a history of IPV, it can be difficult to verbalise it. It is only natural for a therapist to want to be protective and want the client to separate from harm or make a disclosure to safeguard the client. Not doing so is counterintuitive, but that's what some clients need – a safe place to explore and understand what's happening to them. As therapists it is easy to imagine and decide what is the abuse, who may be the victim or the perpetrator, from the initial narrative. It is vital for the client/s to find their space to gain agency to identify abuse, what is right or wrong for them. It is through reflection and feedback of the therapist that clients can begin to see the power and control patterns.

Clients should remain in control of what happens and choose if they wish to make a change or continue to remain in the relationship. There are many repercussions a client faces, and as therapists we have to keep safety in mind. Supervision is useful to balance the judgement of safety. The hardest decision for a therapist is to sit with the client who continues to be abused in the eyes of the therapist. However, if the therapist has reasons to believe that the client and/or partner/s or children may be at serious risk of life or limb by staying in the relationship, they (the therapists) may break the client's confidentiality for protecting life by making a disclosure to relevant authority. It is good practice to always inform the client of this action, but where it is not possible, disclosure should take place with the support of the supervisor and/or insurance guidance. Please note statutory organisations will have specific safeguarding policies which therapists have to follow. Being a witness to the abuse and being able to provide a safe container in the therapy space can help the client make their own decisions. It is vital that the client does not feel judged or shamed.

If leaving the partner is the goal, it must be identified as one by the client as to how and when they would do it. It is not uncommon for the victims of IPV to return to the relationship. It is well documented that if and when they return, they are at higher risk of violence for leaving than before (Home Office, 2021).

I asked how Shaun was coping with everyday life. Whether or not he was able to go to work, make decisions, aware he had choices. I asked him what he felt his choices were? He wanted to make a shift from his position of being trapped. He began to discuss coming out to his family. He wanted to introduce Cara to the family, and then have a discussion with them about his sexuality and choices of partner. He also spoke about meeting up with his friends and explaining to them what has been going on. Earlier Shaun and I discussed the power of support in relationships, and this had sowed the seed for him to reflect on this.

An additional goal can be the identification of a support system for the individual to create resilience and empowerment to take action against the violence or abuse and do it in a way that they are safe, supported and protected. Isolating themselves makes them vulnerable, and so building up a support system can help with self-esteem, reduce isolation, and help them to learn to identify qualities of healthy relationships.

When Shaun was able to establish a way to deal with his abusive relationship, he was able to reflect on his own behaviour and patterns. Some of these behaviours were shameful to Shaun, but when he understood how important they were to protect him at that time, he replaced the shame with compassion. The emotional coercion had left him feeling powerless and trapped.

Challenges facing couples and/or polycules (relationship diversity)

GSRD couples/polycules are forced to go through hoops to adopt children or have IVF and are under scrutiny of social workers as if their parenting skills were lesser than any other general population. They also have to consider bullying and harassment of their children because of having parents who are not cisgender heterosexual. If there are other intersectionalities added, such as colour or race, there are considerable fears GSRD couples have about their children's safety in school and public places. If there is IPV within the relationship, adoption or legitimate surrogacy can be scuppered.

When combined with minority stress, GSRD individuals may be hesitant to admit IPV exists out of fear that their relationship will be held up as a bad example of an already objectionable LGBTQIA+ relationship (Baker et al., 2012; Gehring & Vaske, 2017).

As illustrated with Shaun and Cara, identity concealment and the threat of being outed by an abusive partner go hand-in-hand in IPV. If an individual is not already out to their family, friends, or at work to their co-workers, an abusive partner may use threats to out them as a means of controlling the individual (Gehring & Vaske, 2017). Depending on where the individual works and lives, being outed could result in losing their job, losing their housing, or having other safety concerns.

IPV has not been researched in polyamorous relationships. Whilst polyamorous people have a reputation of being very clear about the boundaries of their relationships, emotions can sometimes take over, and people might not feel grounded in their decision-making. In my experience feelings of jealousy and ownership of partners can often lead to IPV, and this can happen in stealth. Part of the unconscious process may sometimes be due to the negotiation of the relationship between self and others. Identifying attachment styles of individuals can be helpful in understanding the unconscious process, but if IPV does not stop, the client needs to explore if the polyamorous relationship is safe for them or others and what implications it may have in colluding with the partner committing IPV, if they are not the victim.

As it is, it's difficult for GSRD couples or those who are in polycules to have children without being made to feel they are less than their heterosexual other halves. When they are finally able to have children but have IPV in their relationship, they might feel additional responsibility to keep their IPV-entwined relationship going for the sake of the children but also not to let down their friends and family in shame of failing at having a successful relationship with children.

Self-care

Therapists deal with a variety of emotions from clients and themselves. Shame and guilt, grief and loss come to work in a variety of painful, overwhelming and traumatic ways for therapists working with GSRD community. Client deaths, loss of partners through reporting of IPV, death of family members or children, job loss, accidents, and traumatic community loss events all have a major impact on therapists. Ongoing losses related to global public health disasters, suicides, racism and homicides, including killings of trans people, have added to the emotional weight of trauma for therapists. Vicarious trauma can be seen as an occupational hazard, especially when we work with trauma survivors. This term refers to "the cumulative, transformative effect on the provider working with survivors of traumatic life events" (Saakvitne & Pearlman, 1996). Berceli and Napoli (2006) describe vicarious trauma as a change in one's thinking (world view) due to exposure to other people's traumatic stories. Rothschild (2006) offers many insights and suggestions on vicarious trauma in her book *Help for the Helper*.

GSRD clients more often than not seek out GSRD therapists. When working with abuse and violence, the therapist will be exposed to trauma, but working with marginalised and minority clients such as with GSRD community will have added stress and trauma associated with it. In my experience, the stories are hard to hear but harder if the therapist themselves has had similar experience and has a history of abuse and/or violence. Given the prevalence, it is likely that there will be therapists who will be triggered by these stories and need to practise self care, have discussions in supervision and have strategies to support themselves.

Conclusion

On the systemic level, organisations should be fostering an understanding of issues facing the GSRD community, their needs, and aspects of IPV unique to LGBTQIA+ individuals (Ford et al., 2013). All trainings should include information on how to use GSRD-inclusive language, power dynamics in GSRD relationships, and a discussion of concerns faced by advocates in order to address those concerns and overcome obstacles that may keep GSRD individuals from reaching out for support. If you are a therapist who is in contact with organisations that may support GSRD clients, you may wish to ensure they are GSRD aware to support these clients. Organisations that provide such training can be found on the Galop website (galop.org.uk).

References

1   Abbott, J., Johnson, R., Koziol-McLain, J., & Lowenstein, S. R. (1995, June 14). Domestic violence against women. Incidence and prevalence in an emergency department population. *JAMA*, *273*(22), 1763–1767. http://doi.org/10.1001/jama.273.22.1763

2   Baker, N., Buick, J., Kim, S., Moniz, S., & Nava, K. (2012). Lessons from examining same-sex intimate partner violence. *Sex Roles*, *69*(4), 182–192.

3   Barker, M. J., & Gabb, J. (2016). *The Secrets of Enduring Love: How to Make Relationships Last*. London: Vermilion.

4   Berceli, D., & Napoli, M. A. (2006). Proposal for a mindfulness-based trauma prevention program for social work professionals. *Complementary Health Practice Review*, *11*(3), 153–165. http://doi.org/10.1177/1533210106297989

5   Brown, T. N. T., & Herman, J. L. (2015). *Intimate Partner Violence and Sexual Abuse Among LGBT People*. A review of existing research. UCLA. School of Law. Williams Institute. Retrieved from https://williamsinstitute.law.ucla.edu/publications/ipv-sex-abuse-lgbt-people/

6   Campbell, J. C., Anderson, J. C., McFadgion, A., Gill, J., Zink, E., Patch, M., Callwood, G., & Campbell, D. (2018, June). The effects of intimate partner violence and probable traumatic brain injury on central nervous system symptoms. *Journal of Women's Health*, *27*(6), 761–767. http://doi.org/10.1089/jwh.2016.6311

7   Campbell, J. C., & Soeken, K. L. (1999). Forced sex and intimate partner violence: Effects on women's risk and women's health. *Violence Against Women*, *5*(9), 1017–1035. http://doi.org/10.1177/1077801299005009003

8   Carvalho, A. F., Lewis, R. J., Derlega, V. J., Winstead, B. A., & Viggiano, C. (2011). Internalized sexual minority stressors and same-sex intimate partner violence. *Journal of Family Violence*, *26*, 501–509. https://doi.org/10.1007/s10896-011-9384-2

9   Cavacuiti, C., & Chan, E. (2008). Gay abuse screening protocol (GASP): Screening for abuse in gay male relationships. *Journal of Homosexuality*, *54*, 423–438.

10 Chrisler, J. C., & Ferguson, S. (2006). Violence against women as a public health issue. *Annals of the New York Academy of Sciences*, *1087*(1), 235–249. https://doi.org/10.1196/ANNALS.1385.009

11 Coker, A., Davis, K., Arias, I., Desai, S., Sanderson, M., Brandt, H., & Smith, P. (2002). Physical and mental health effects of intimate partner violence for men and women. *American Journal of Preventive Medicine*, *23*, 260–268. https://doi.org/10.1016/j.amepre.2021.10.001

12 CPS. (2022). Pre-trial therapy. *Legal Guidance*. Retrieved from www.cps.gov.uk/legal-guidance/pre-trial-therapy

13 Davies, D., & Neal, C. (1996). *Pink Therapy. A Guide for Counsellors and Therapists Working with Lesbian, Gay and Bisexual Clients*. Berkshire: Open University Press.

14 Donovan, C., & Hester, M. (2010). 'I hate the word "victim"': An exploration of recognition of domestic violence in same sex relationships. *Social Policy and Society*, *9*(2), 279–289. https://doi.org/10.1017/S1474746409990406

15 Ford, C. L., Hilton, K. L., Holt, S. L., & Slavin, T. (2013). Intimate partner violence prevention services and resources in Los Angeles: Issues, needs challenges for assisting lesbian, gay, bisexual and transgender clients. *Health Promotion Practice*, *14*, 841–849.

16 Gehring, K. S., & Vaske, J. C. (2017). Out in the open: The consequences of intimate partner violence for victims in same-sex and opposite-sex relationships. *Journal of Interpersonal Violence*, *32*(23), 3669–3692. https://doi.org/10.1177/0886260515600877

17 Home Office. (2013). *Definition of Domestic Violence and Abuse: Guide for Local Areas*. Retrieved from www.gov.uk/government/publications/definition-of-domestic-violence-and-abuse-guide-for-local-areas

18   Home Office. (2021). *Domestic Abuse: How to Get Help*. Retrieved from www.gov. uk/guidance/domestic-abuse-how-to-get-help

19   Hubbard, L. (2021). *The Hate Crime Report 2021: Supporting LGBT+ Victims of Hate Crime, London, Galop*. Retrieved from https://galop.org.uk/wp-content/ uploads/2021/06/Galop-Hate-Crime-Report-2021-1.pdf

20   Iantaffi, A. (2021). *Gender Trauma. Healing Cultural, Social, and Historical Gendered Trauma*. London: Jessica Kingsley Publishers.

21   Jülich, S. (2005). Stockholm syndrome and child sexual abuse. *Journal of child sexual abuse, 14*(3), 107–129. Retrieved from https://www.noos.org.br/carloszuma/Shirley%20Julich/Julich%20-%20Stockholm%20Syndrome.pdf

22   Karakurt, G., Whiting, K., Jones, S. E., Lowe, M. J., & Rao, S. M. (2021, October 5). Brain injury and mental health among the victims of intimate partner violence: A caseseries exploratory study. *Frontiers in Psychology, 12*, 710602. http://doi.org/10.3389/fpsyg.2021.710602

23   Kozlowski, L. (2020). *Trauma Bonding: Understanding and Overcoming the Traumatic Bond in a Narcissistic Relationship*. Escape the Narcissist. Retrieved from https://escapethenarcissist.com

24   Langenderfer-Magruder, L., Whitfield, D. L., Walls, N. E., Kattari, S. K., & Ramos, D. (2016). Experiences of intimate partner violence and subsequent police reporting among lesbian, gay, bisexual, transgender, and queer adults in Colorado: Comparing rates of cisgender and transgender victimization. *Journal of Interpersonal Violence, 31*(5), 855–871. http://doi.org/10.1177/0886260514556767

25   Machado, C. M. (2020). *In the Dream House*. Minneapolis, MN: Graywolf Press.

26   Meyer, I. H., & Northridge, M. E. (Eds.). (2007). *The Health of Sexual Minorities: Public Health Perspectives on Lesbian, Gay, Bisexual and Transgender Populations*. New York: Springer.

27   Penone, G., & Guarnaccia, C. (2018). Intimate partner violence within same sex couples: A qualitative review of the literature from a psychodynamic perspective. *International Journal of Psychoanalysis and Education, 10*(1), 32–46.

28   Rothschild, B. (2006). *Help for the Helper. Self-Care Strategies for Managing Burnout and Stress*. New York: W.W. Norton & Co.

29   Saakvitne, K. W., & Pearlman, L. A. (1996). *Transforming the Pain: A Workbook on Vicarious Traumatization*. Traumatic Stress Inst, Ctr for Adult & Adolescent Psychotherapy, LLC. New York, NY: W.W. Norton & Co.

30   SaveLives Report. (2018). *Free to Be Safe LGBT+ People Experiencing Domestic Abuse*. Retrieved from https://safelives.org.uk/sites/default/files/resources/Free%20 to%20be%20safe%20web.pdf

31   Shahbaz, C., & Chirinos, P. (2017). *Becoming a Kink Aware Therapist*. Abingdon: Routledge.

32   Stonewall. (2018). LGBT in Britain. *Home and Communities*. Retrieved from www. stonewall.org.uk/sites/default/files/lgbt_in_britain_home_and_communities.pdf

33   Taylor, N. T. B., & Herman, J. L. (2015). Intimate partner violence and sexual abuse among LGBT people – A review of existing research. *The Williams Institute*. Retrieved from https://williamsinstitute.law.ucla.edu/publications/ipv-sex-abuse-lgbt-people/

34   Thompson, R. (2021). *Rough: How Violence Has Found Its Way into the Bedroom and What We Can Do about It*. Square Peg. London: Penguin Random House.

35   UK Government: Domestic abuse Act. (2021). Retrieved from www.legislation.gov. uk/ukpga/2021/17/contents/enacted

36 UK Government: Sexual Offences Act. (2003). Retrieved from www.legislation.gov. uk/ukpga/2003/42/contents

37 World Health Organization (WHO). (2012). *Understanding and Addressing Violence Against Women.* Retrieved from https://apps.who.int/iris/bitstream/ handle/10665/77432/WHO_RHR_12.36_eng.pdf

Chapter 9

Exploring the impact of a religious background or identity on LGBTQ people

Saquib Ahmad

Fore note and acknowledgements

This chapter was written using three case studies, from structured interviews and social media surveys. The identities of all who are mentioned here have been deliberately changed to protect those who volunteered their time, provided consent for information sharing and allowed their therapeutic journeys to be published. I thank you all with my uttermost gratitude. It is with your truths that I have been able to complete this chapter and provide some guidance to working with LGBTQ people who have a religious background or identity.

Introduction

To have or have had a religious identity or background and to be of the LGBTQ community is not without its own unique intersectional challenges. It has been evidenced (Boppana & Gross, 2019) that many may develop internalised homo-negativity/homophobia (IH) as a consequence of these identities. IH has been associated with reduced relationship quality in same-sex relationships, leading to an impact on relationship satisfaction, commitment, and intimacy (Thies et al., 2016). This chapter will explore how LGBTQ people of religious backgrounds, specifically Christian, Jewish, and Muslim faiths, experience key difficulties due to their intersectional identities, how they cope with what on the surface can be very opposing identities, and what professionals can do to help these individuals improve their mental well-being when they seek support.

For the purpose of this chapter, religiosity is defined as the relationship one has with various behavioural aspects of one's religion, for example, praying, reading religious texts, attending religious institutes, partaking in religious festivals, etc., with the assumption that there is belief or faith in the foundations of the religion, irrespective of engagement in the previously mentioned behaviours.

Ben – gay, Jewish, white male (mid 30s)

Ben is a British, gay cis male, born in North London. He describes himself and his family as culturally Jewish thus having a moderate level of religiosity. The

DOI: 10.4324/9781003260561-10

family celebrates all Jewish festivals, they partake in the weekly Sabbath, and growing up he remembers going to a few synagogues till the family settled on one which matched their religiosity but also their inclusive attitudes. He states there were openly gay and lesbian members of the congregation who were liked and respected by his family and others in the community, thus Ben's coming out was somewhat less difficult than some Jewish people born in a more Orthodox setting.

Sexually, Ben often struggled to be "satisfied" due to his dislike of the uncircumcised penis. This meant he did not enjoy giving oral sex to his partners who often were uncircumcised. He felt more comfortable and more aroused by those who were circumcised like him. Male circumcision is a religious requirement for those of Jewish and Muslim faith. Outside of religious obligations, male infants in the USA are routinely circumcised, and 'uncut' penises are often understood to be ugly (Allan, 2018). Ben, therefore, found himself preferring 'cut' men that he would meet whilst travelling for work and/or pleasure in the USA, or Muslim men and other Jewish men, commenting on the aesthetics and the hygiene component of same-sex sex.

Furthermore, when dating non-Jewish men, Ben felt there was a relational distance due to the lack of understanding and acceptance of his religiosity. Ben was criticised by his white-British, non-Jewish partners when he was unwilling to go out on Saturday nights due to observing Sabbath with his family or prioritising religious ceremonies. It is not uncommon for minority LGBTQ people to experience racism in the form of overt racism, or covert racism in the form of microaggressions, and unconscious biases (Balsam et al., 2011; McConnell et al., 2018) which can cause mental health problems. Ben felt he was judged by many he dated for practicing his religion.

During his mid-20s, Ben relocated to Israel, where he met his current partner who matched many of the characteristics of assortative mating (Buss, 1985), including, race, religion, socioeconomic status, age, physical characteristics and personality. Ben also felt being in this society where his religiosity and sexuality are respected and supported helped him sustain his relationship.

Ben's case highlights that, though not the only factor, religiosity matching played a crucial part in the ongoing success of their relationship.

Denia – lesbian, Greek Orthodox, white female (early 30s)

Denia is the youngest of two sisters born into a Greek Orthodox family in Greece. She remembers religion having a big influence on her upbringing. Her mother and grandmothers were more religious than her father and grandparents though both sexes of the different generations had a common minimum baseline "like most Greeks". The family also went to church and prayed together.

She recalled that her family were openly homophobic. There were frequent homophobic comments of openly gay people and those who displayed non-gender confirming behaviours, for example, women not marrying, or men being effeminate. She knew what the expectations of her were and followed them.

She experienced her first same-sex experience at university and at the time did not associate it with being a lesbian or even bisexual; she rationalised it at the time as an isolated incident. Models of sexual orientation identity propose the following developmental stages:

1   Questioning one's heterosexuality is accompanied by acute distress and fear about being 'found out', which is coupled with low self-esteem and self-doubt in reference to being different.
2   Responses to dissolve these feelings which can either lead to openness and self-acceptance or responses which lead to identity foreclosure or compartmentalisation of public and private aspects of the identity.

(Floyd & Stein, 2002)

For Denia it was the latter; her sexual exploration with another girl was not a public affair but something private and not relevant for others to know, which was the opposite to how her friends at the time behaved around their individual sexual experiences.

Denia was only able to 'come out' as a lesbian when she felt she was more independent of her parent's control and influence and had assumed her sexual identity further. This is in line with research on sexual identity self-disclosure; coming out earlier is associated with greater independence from parental oversight and the type of peer pressure one may experience in high school. Delayed acceptance was also associated with delayed disclosure to family and siblings, historical use of substances and higher levels of internalised and perceived homophobia (Ong et al., 2021).

Denia remembered feeling she could not accept herself as there was so much homophobia around her, and at the same time she dreamed of getting more independence away from her family and environmental stressors so she could be free.

After university Denia relocated to London, meeting more LGBTQ peers. She started to become more confident in herself, and her self-acceptance grew. However, she still carried some shame which inevitably bled into her relationships as she held the core belief that she was 'bad' and this could not be changed because she could not become straight and would ultimately go to hell in accordance with her religious beliefs.

Schema therapy states that due to noxious life experiences, one can develop negative core beliefs such as 'I am bad', 'I am weak', I am not good enough', and so on, and due to the shame elicited by activation of these beliefs, individuals cope by using three broad coping strategies:

1   Clear avoidance of situations that may activate the schema (schema avoidance).
2   Using strategies to go over and above to disprove the schema (schema overcompensation).

3   When the individual is not able to use the previous two strategies, they are forced to face certain situations and yield to the schema (schema surrender).

Despite Denia's core belief, she was able to have relationships, unlike many with similar experiences, however inadvertently either found partners that were unsuitable for her (schema avoidance) or she would sabotage the relationship (schema surrender), thus always maintaining the belief she was 'bad' (Young et al., 2003).

Zahid – bisexual, Muslim, British Pakistani male (mid 30s)

Zahid was born in Pakistan and raised in the UK by his single mother. He is the youngest of three siblings and noticed his attraction to same-sex people around the age of nine.

He was born into a middle-class Pakistani household from his paternal side, which housed his own immediate family, his grandparents, other relatives, and their nuclear families.

He described his family's religiosity using the term "Deen aur Dunya", loosely translating to the art of balancing faith and religiosity (deen) and day-to-day life and worldliness (dunya). He described his family as "fairly progressive" and open minded for Pakistani standards but still very religious, which he stated was typical of this class of Lahori-ites (people from the Pakistani city of Lahore).

Zahid found moving to the UK at the age of seven difficult as his social and emotional support network shrank from over twenty people to three overnight, which now only included his mother, brother, and sister as his parents separated. Zahid's mother became emotionally unavailable to him as she worked two jobs, and the priority now was to provide rather than nurture, causing him to feel abandoned by everyone and believing he was a 'bad boy'.

In his teenage years he became more aware of sexual feelings, though he did not have a word for bisexuality at this point. He knew what it meant to be gay and straight. Bisexuality was not a concept he ever considered for himself. He noticed homophobia in school. Zahid was aware he had certain qualities which were considered feminine and associated with being gay. He was sometimes teased, being insulted with homophobic slurs such as "fag" or "queer". Though Zahid would say he was somewhat popular and generally liked, he did recognise and state that he did not always have it easy, and he had to a "play a role". This masculinity policing is a form of homophobia which is laced in misogyny (Kimmel, 2003); the two go hand in hand.

As an attempt to run away from stressors at home and his surrounding and to gain independence, Zahid left his home city to go to university as far away as he could. Here he could start afresh, and he could explore his sexuality safely. Zahid had his first date with a man and fell in love and finally came out to a few selected friends as bisexual. Within a couple of years he also came out to his mother as bisexual. He believed he was pretending to be bisexual as this would ultimately justify to his gay friends why he would get married to a woman and to his family that he can be like his siblings and be "normal and acceptable". Zahid had IH, but he also had biphobia. He, at the core of himself, did not believe bisexuality existed, even though he had been sexually active with men and women and had felt sexually satisfied by both.

Biphobia, unlike homophobia, may exist because of the ongoing debate around how to conceptualise this sexual orientation, whether that be through the Kinsey scale, where heterosexuality is measured against homosexuality with extremes being on either end of a continuum as anchor points (Kinsey et al., 1948), or through Storms (1980) separate dimensions theory where heterosexuality and homosexuality are on two separate dimensions and a bisexual is high in both dimensions of heterosexuality and homosexuality. This confusion around the conceptualisation rather than validating of the sexual orientation of bisexuals may be a reason for the existence of biphobia.

Zahid remembers his gay friends making jokes about bisexuals, commenting "Bi today, gay tomorrow" referring to bisexuality as a transitional sexuality (MacDonald, 1981). He himself mocked those whom he deemed to be "too gay" to be bisexual, which relates to the Kinsey's scaling of sexuality. Zahid took to the Quran and Islamic literature which clearly categorised gay men, lesbian women, and trans-people but did not mention bisexuals, which further added to his biphobia.

Due to religious cultural pressures he experienced; he made the conscious decision to get married in his mid-20s. The marriage was short-lived for several factors but one which overarched them all; the belief that bisexuals are denying their true homosexual nature. He further confirmed this to himself by his extra-marital affairs with other men. His love and his sexual/romantic attraction for his wife, and general attraction to other women, was in competition with his internalised biphobia, which was too strong to withstand any information that challenged it. Information was distorted and discarded, and those around him fed into this narrative thus maintaining his internalised biphobia (IBP).

Zahid had several experiences of psychotherapy following his divorce to deal with the trauma of the breakdown of his marriage and the underlying issues this opened up for him. His post-divorce counselling caused significant damage. Zahid believed his therapist implied that he was also denying his true homosexual orientation and that he only got married to continue to play this role of 'straight man'. Years later, Zahid was courageous to seek therapy again, this time with a knowledgeable clinician who provided psycho-education on sexual orientations. This challenged Zahid's internalised biphobia and pointed out to him the inconsistencies he was avoiding facing, which served the purpose to maintain the belief that he was "bad", because why else would a gay man marry a straight woman and cause her so much pain?

It is important to note that Zahid's IH stemmed from his environment, like for many others, and although his immediate family did not directly condemn or disapprove of homosexuality, they did not approve of it either. It was more an unsaid knowledge he acquired. However, his biphobia developed more through the exposure to biphobic narratives that existed within the gay community which he was a part of, the lack of bi-visibility, and the absence of bisexuality within Islamic literature he took to.

Mulick (1999) identified that biphobia exists in heterosexual and homosexual communities. He also identified some evidence of the prevalence of IBP. Biphobia amongst gay men is an example of double discrimination where bisexuals experience discrimination from heterosexuals and gay communities (Bennett, 1992), which may explain the lack of bi-visibility Zahid experienced.

Through regular psychotherapy, exposure to literature and other bisexuals, Zahid was able to work on his IBP and become more accepting of himself. Zahid began to date women again, which he stopped following his divorce due to shame associated with how he believed he 'cheated' his wife with his sexuality, and was now open to them about his sexuality from the get-go and would educate friends and family on their biphobic attitudes and its impact. He further consolidated his religious beliefs by understanding that bi-visibility, though lacking in the Quran, is not so lacking in Islamic history with many prominent Mughal emperors to Islamic philosophers displaying sexual fluidity and not being defined in absolute categories such as straight, gay, or bisexual.

Sexual identity

Our identity is shaped by many factors, including our family, religion, ethnic culture, race, sexuality, gender, age, political beliefs, generation, and so on.

It is not uncommon for LGBTQ people who also have a religious identity to struggle with the two identities, which can lead to mental health problems (Boppana & Gross, 2019). A study on 144 gay Israeli men demonstrated that severe identity conflicts led to poorer mental health (Zeidner & Zevulun, 2017), as homophobia and gender normative beliefs have been highly prevalent culturally in most major religious communities. Whether or not sexual and gender 'deviations' are permissible is up for interpretation depending on what text you read, which cleric you speak to, or how your family introduced religion to you.

It is also important to note that cultural norms, practices, and interpretations of texts of one religious community compared to another can vary, producing nuances to how homosexuality and gender non-conforming behaviours are seen and treated. This may either pave a way for identity consolidation or identity conflicts as demonstrated by the discussed case studies.

I used social media (Instagram) to ask LGBTQ people of religious backgrounds two questions:

1   Growing up did you have access to a religious environment (at home, place of worship and or other) where you felt you were or could be accepted as a LGBTQ person? Yes or No?
2   If you had access to a religious environment (at home, place of worship and or other) growing up which was more accepting of LGBTQ people, do you

believe this would have had a positive impact on your religiosity (any behaviour, physical or mental towards the religion)? Yes or no?

The survey of 68 LGBTQ people demonstrated that only 21% of the participants had access to a religious environment where they felt accepted as an LGBTQ person, and 73% went further to say that had their environments been more LGBTQ accepting, they believe that it would have impacted on their religiosity positively. Though this survey by no means is a large sample and participant contribution was not controlled in any way, it does shed some light on the importance of cultivating dual identities. If the 73% had access to the LGBTQ inclusive environments, they may, for instance, have prayed more, gone to a place of worship more, read more religious texts, thought about God more, talked to others about religion more, and so on. It can be inferred that the inclusivity of a religious environment to LGBTQ people has an impact on the religiosity of those LGBTQ people in contact with it. Furthermore, we could hypothesise that this may impact on the reconciliation and/or integration of the different parts of one's identity (religious identity and LGBTQ identity) should there be inclusivity of LGBTQ people in the religious environments.

Despite the presence of this traditional value, it can generally be said that over the generations there has been much progress made in attitudes towards LGBTQ people across Western Europe and North America, bringing us into the 'Gay marriage generation' with progressive changes in laws increasing the rights of LGBTQ people and decreasing discrimination through equal rights laws. These generational shifts would inevitably also impact religious communities, be it at varying degrees, with some communities being more tolerant and welcoming of LGBTQ people than others.

We see examples of religious communities in Europe interpreting and practicing religion in various ways. Seyran Ates, a human rights lawyer, founder and Imam of Ibn Rushd-Goeth Mosque in Berlin, welcomes LGBTQ people. Ates is breaking gender norms in mainstream Islamic practices by being a female Imam who leads women *and* men into prayer and promotes the inclusion of sexual and gender minorities into a mosque, who otherwise would be invisible in such environments, creating a new paradigm for German-Muslim-LGBTQ people.

In London, the St Mary's Church, which represents Church of England welcomes LGBTQ people as individuals and as couples. Its LGBTQ members also serve the church by leading in Sunday services. Though at present they do not perform same-sex marriages or blessings, St Mary's has already gone ahead of many churches around the world.

Here you have two established religious communities breaking traditional norms around LGBTQ topics by becoming more inclusive. In parallel to this, there are LGBTQ communities who have established their own religious subcommunities. In the UK alone we have several faith-based LGBTQ associations, including Imaan, an association founded in 1999 in London, which offers support meetings and faith activities for Muslims who identify as LGBTQ and those who are questioning; Gay Christian Europe, which focuses on LGBTQ Christians, providing groups, welcoming churches and resources local to them, online and in person; and also the Jewish LGBTQ+ group, founded in 1972, functioning from St John's Wood, which is the longest established Jewish LGBTQ group in the world.

The formation of these progressive and inclusive subcommunities may serve to provide the acceptance, validation, and normalisation that many otherwise may not have from their immediate families, relatives, colleagues, friends, and traditional religious environments which can aid to consolidate religious and sexual identities, thus decreasing mental health problems in LGBTQ people of less progressive religious backgrounds.

The three case studies highlight how a religious background can impact one's view of self in relation to sexuality in varying ways depending on the messages received from their environments. For Ben, the exposure to sexual diversity his parents invited into his life by changing synagogues allowed Ben to have a higher level of self-acceptance as he was able to see a place for his sexual identity within a religious environment where sexual diversity was accepted and normalised. This external acceptance and normalisation lowered his levels of IH, and so he was able to self-disclose to his parents much earlier than Denia and Zahid, and subsequently have relationships that were more suited to his overall identity and needs.

Zahid in contrast came out as bisexual sooner than Denia and so was able to address his IH (though not his IBP) sooner than Denia. This perhaps can be explained by Western Europe being somewhat more progressive towards LGBTQ issues than Southern Europe, coupled with the parental independence he had by moving away sooner and the "fairly progressive" family he came from.

It would be interesting to hypothesise how the three individuals' sexual identities would develop had they been born in an earlier generation where there was less progression in LGBTQ issues compared to their millennial context of coming to sexual maturity and ultimately coming out. Bitterman and Hess (2020) demonstrate that LGBTQ people unlike their heterosexual counterparts relate not only to their birth generation but also their sexual maturing and subsequent coming out generations. Therefore it is likely to influence the ease at which LGBTQ people of a religious background would be able to consolidate their identities.

Zahid's later acceptance of his bisexuality coincides with Generation Z's generational shift in their attitudes towards bisexuality. The validity of bisexuals by this generation through the use of social media may have also had some influence on Zahid's IBP and therefore allow him to address conscious and unconscious behaviours which reinforced it.

Ben sustained his religiosity throughout, so much so that he immigrated to Israel to further consolidate his intersectional identities (being gay and Jewish), which he felt was difficult to do in the UK. On the other hand, Denia grew an aversion to religion and the cultural practices around it, which subsequently led to a decrease in her religiosity until eventually in her mid 20s, she became an Atheist. Being permanently based in London was helpful for her mental well-being and made her more self-accepting as there was not a constant reminder from family members that God would punish her. She also noticed this helped her relationship with her family as she felt her need for their acceptance decreased.

Relationships and sex

Individuals in positive relationships have been found to have a reduced risk of depression, anxiety, and suicidal ideation, where negative relationships have shown to have the opposite effect (Santini et al., 2015).

The shame that one experiences can have a significant impact on one's relationship. Even today, LGBTQ people experience a lot of discrimination. These covert and/or overt assaults on individuals and a community as a whole can have long-lasting consequences, which will inevitably leak into the sex and relationships these individuals have. In my 14 years of practice and interactions with patients, friends, and family who identify as LGBTQ, many often comment on the difficulties which they feel are inherent to LGBTQ relationships. I stress the importance of compassion for oneself and other LGBTQ people as often *we* do not always have access to role models to base relationships on and have often not fully processed the inherent difficulties that come with being a sexual and/ or gender minority. Thus, two individuals attempt to dance their unsynchronised tango with many toes that are stubbed in the process. The context in which these individuals may emerge and come together is often riddled with challenges due to the overt and covert discrimination LGBTQ people still experience.

LGBTQ couples may experience some challenges in achieving certain relationship milestones compared to heterosexual couples in emerging adults. For instance, youths who are not engaged in LGBTQ social networks found it harder to identify prospective partners and have access to information about LGBTQ relationships compared to those who had access (Eyre et al., 2007). Another study showed how differing levels of outness slowed relationship progression and caused relationship distress, for example, a delayed start in sexual activity and pretending to be friends in public, respectively (Patterson et al., 2013). Where Ben was able to identify a prospective partner with somewhat ease as an emerging adult, Denia struggled, and when she did meet someone, her negative attitudes towards her sexual orientation due to her faith made it difficult to be open, putting pressure on the relationship.

A study on the mental health of Jewish gay men in Israel also demonstrated that those in relationships had better mental health than single, gay Jewish men. However, men with severe identity conflicts reported poorer mental health (Zeidner & Zevulun, 2017). Ben saw a decrease in his experience of minority stress (Meyer, 1995) by immigrating to Israel. Although his gay identity made him a minority amongst the heterosexual majority, living in Tel Aviv was empowering as the progressive attitudes towards LGBTQ communities of the city made it a haven in a highly religious and politicised country. He could embrace both his Jewish and gay identities freely.

Zahid's IBP prevented him from ever being secure in any relationship, same-sex or different-sex; when he was with a woman, he believed he was gay and pretending to be bisexual, and when he was with a man, he felt his male partners judge his bisexuality irrespective of his own judgements towards his sexuality. Zahid also experienced occasional unreliable erections; on deeper exploration he discovered this was his own insecurity about himself. With women this insecurity confirmed he was *actually* gay, and with men he justified it as he did not like the person enough, instead of thinking more compassionately about himself.

Considerations for therapy

The therapeutic relationship is consistently shown to be a strong predictor for positive outcomes within therapy outweighing therapeutic discipline and interventions (Safran et al., 2011; Gaztambide, 2012; Martin et al., 2000). However, the relationship itself cannot be considered a rigid concept that remains unchanged once it has been established, and like any relationship, it is susceptible to ruptures.

When working with LGBTQ patients, it is essential to have knowledge, understanding, skill, and confidence in working with people from such diverse communities. Often a lack of the above leads to ruptures and therefore disengagement.

> Being Muslim and queer is hard enough without a shrink making you feel bad. My therapist didn't understand why it was difficult to simply be open. She didn't understand why it was important to have support from my family and be myself too – She simply made me feel that I was too weak to be me.
>
> Shabaz 38 – Queer, British Pakistani Muslim

It is suggested that North American and Western European psychology, which continues to dominate the work of psychology, is driven by ten basic factors: individuality, reductionism, experiment-based empiricism, scientism, quantification/measurement, materialism, male dominance, objectivity, nomothetic laws, and rationality. These assumptions can be in direct conflict with the worldviews and praxiological assumptions derived from them, of cultures that are not North American and Western European (Marsella, 2009).

Shabaz's experience illustrates the clear conflict between worldviews around individual independence versus parental dependence. Kumaraswamy (2007) claimed that a certain amount of dependence on parents is normal in Malay culture, and efforts to instil absolute autonomy by a mental health professional would cause more harm than good as this is a Western standard. This is applicable to many non-Western cultures who, despite residing in Europe, hold conflicting values.

Furthermore, the negative consequences of coming out can be very real in some extreme cases, where individuals may face physical danger. It is the job of the professional to help the patient assess these dangers and create safety plans if they wish to come out to such families and/or communities. Where this imminent threat is not the case, other consequences should also be considered, such as emotional abuse, verbal abuse, neglect, or financial abuse, and it is important to ensure some plans are made to help manage these issues, including corresponding with appropriate agencies where necessary, such as adult or child social care services, GPs, and the police.

> My therapist was an Atheist, I know it shouldn't matter but it bothered me as I just didn't want to explain myself.
>
> Edward 26 – gay, Catholic, Caribbean Black male

Therapist matching is an issue of much psychological debate with evidence in support of it and evidence suggesting it does not matter. Abernethy and Lancia (1998) demonstrate that a lack of religious training or heritage may lead to therapists avoiding discussions around the topic, whereas those with a religious background in their openness to religion may overemphasise its importance at the expense of other important patient communications. They suggest four principles to consider in order to effectively work with religious content: (1) degree of openness, (2) attunement, (3) consultation, and (4) interpretation.

Through my own personal practice, I believe another important principle is curiosity, as patients can sometimes feel there is no room to talk about a religious identity within the context of therapy. We are often able to be curious about certain emissions in therapy relating to the patient's identity, for example, their sexuality, ethnicity, or education, but due to our own beliefs about therapy, we may avoid asking explicitly about the presence of a religious identity.

Therapists' awareness of their potential automatic responses to avoid or even not consider religious content is an important prerequisite to working with this content. Becoming more aware of these reactions will allow therapists to counter them so that they can attend appropriately to their patients' communications or non-communications, for example, a practicing gay Muslim not talking about the impact of the two identities.

A common problem that arises in the attempt to reduce distress within religious-LGBTQ people in regard to their religious beliefs and sexual identity is to elicit compassion from a dogmatic perspective with comments such as, "My understanding is that (insert religion) is a faith of compassion with God being the most merciful". As well-intentioned as this may be, it can cause frustration in the individual who may see the therapist as naïve and unknowledgeable to religious texts, especially in reference to the story of Sodom and Gomorrah or its Muslim equivalent People of the Prophet Lot, which are widely used in Abrahamic religions to justify the sin inherent to 'practicing homosexuality'.

Instead, it may be more helpful to encourage patients to explore alternative interpretations of religious texts and speak to religious clerics who interpret religious texts in an alternative way. Though little, there is at least some literature in this field, thus providing an alternative narrative and allowing some room for consolidation in the patient's internal conflict. It is not uncommon for religious-LGBTQ patients to be highly avoidant to such information prior to therapy or even be unaware that it exists. Kugle (2010), in his book, provides an alternative reflection on Muslim gay, lesbian, and transgender people.

Part of homework as per behavioural therapies, patients can be encouraged to seek out and meet peers. The acquisition of a supportive social network is vital (Floyd & Stein, 2002). In the earlier cases, the social networks both acquired by Ben and Denia provided appropriate social support related to their intersectional identities, Jewish-gay and Greek-lesbian, which neither felt they could get in their respective birth countries. For Zahid, having access to new bi-inclusive information as well as new social networks aided his journey.

In 2011 Ayatollah Ali al-Sistani, the most prominent Shia Leader, renounced the fatwa on the killing of gay people from his website following weeks of talks with the London office of an Iraqi gay and lesbian organisation (Howden, 2011). This demonstrates some potential changes in the commonly upheld narratives around Islam and homosexuality. Sign posting patients to LGBTQ inclusive religious organisations (progressive churches, synagogues, or mosques) or subcommunities which provide a 'Brave space', like Imaan, may help with this process of identity consolidation through socio-religious validation of their identities in this case. Generational shifts in religious communities may be taking place which they are not aware of.

> Our couple's therapist constantly pathologised my needs and normalised his. She did this by telling me we are from different cultures and religions and so I cannot expect from him things which I deemed important in a relationship and inversely would normalise his expectations of me which he deemed important in a relationship – the message I got was clear, my culture and values are the problem, his are the solution.
>
> Saquib 33 – British, Pakistani, bisexual Muslim

As mentioned earlier, psychology today predominantly holds a Western worldview and thus, more often than not, is practised and taught from this perspective. Western therapies therefore have depended on and upheld the dominant discourse (White-Christian-heterosexual values) and reinforced the marginalisation of statements and practices which exist outside of the dominant representation in society. This can cause therapists and interracial couples or couples of different religions to consciously or unconsciously collude with one another, leading to certain discourses being avoided, dismissed, or minimised at the expense of others (Nardi et al., 2012).

When working with interracial couples or couples of different religions, research suggests that narrative approaches may be more suitable than traditional couple therapy approaches. Its focus on telling and understanding stories may help the aligning of couples with one another because when one partner is telling their story, it may be easier for the other to align with the protagonist and the story, which could lead to an increase in understanding and empathy (Kim et al., 2012).

Like any form of discrimination, racism, anti-Semitism, Islamophobia, Xenophobia, and other forms of discrimination towards people of colour, religious and ethnic minorities are part of British and European society, and to avoid it or minimise its impact simply helps to maintain them. It is not uncommon for those who experience these issues to avoid talking about them and minimise its impact, as minorities have also been conditioned to protect the status quo. It is helpful to explore these issues with your patients as they may not have discussed the inherent difficulties of minority distress and may not have the words to attach their experiences and feelings to concepts such as white fragility, intersectionality, and gaslighting, which are modern concepts that our patients may not be familiar with.

Like others, LGBTQ religious people also cope with their identity conflicts with the use of cognitive dissonance (Festinger, 1962), where the distress caused by two conflicting concepts, feelings, or beliefs is managed by distortion of the information, thus eliminating the conflict and distress, for example, "this is a carrot cake, carrots are healthy, so the cake is not bad for my diet". Identifying the strategy in itself can be illuminating and thus paves the way to undercovering other instances where the individual may do this.

Conclusions

Like any community, LGBTQ people are not a monolith. There are myriad representations that form subcommunities. LGBTQ people of religious background or identity also form such subcommunities, and individuals will have varying degrees of religiosity from very high to none.

When working with these individuals or couples, it is essential for therapists to be aware of their own views, assumptions, and beliefs about same-sex relationships, gender non-conformativity, misogyny, racism, xenophobia, anti-Semitism, Islamophobia, secularism, transphobia, biphobia, homophobia, and other discriminatory attitudes as it is normal for all of us to have such attitudes or biases to some extent due to the systems in which we live in, study in, work in, and vote into; therefore, these biases will inevitably present themselves consciously or unconsciously in our sessions. The minority stress that LGBTQ people of religious identities and backgrounds experience can make them highly sensitive to these conscious or unconscious displays.

These subcommunities can experience rejection on a human level but also on a spiritual level due to their teachings around their identity. This can create a profound sense of fear in emerging individuals worrying about their afterlife and thus the need to compartmentalise the identities or avoid huge parts of their identity. This is a common practice until they learn to consolidate their identities and make peace with themselves, with the support of an open, empathic, and inquisitive therapist. If long-term therapy is not possible, phased-based approaches to therapy may be an alternative with therapy breaks (1–3 months) between phases. It can take months and even years depending on the damage done by their perceived or actual rejection from their respective religions and/or cultures and environments.

It is not for us to decide whether their religiosity should be increased or decreased, nor whether they should even need a religion. It is our job to help them find ways to accept their identities, allowing them to thrive and not simply survive.

References

Abernethy, A. D., & Lancia, J. J. (1998). Religion and the psychotherapeutic relationship. Transferential and countertransferential dimensions. *The Journal of Psychotherapy Practice and Research, 7*(4), 281–289.

Allan, J. A. (2018). The foreskin aesthetic or ugliness reconsidered. *Men and Masculinities*, 1097184X1775303. http://doi.org/10.1177/1097184x17753038

Balsam, K. F., Molina, Y., Beadnell, B., Simoni, J., & Walters, K. (2011). Measuring multiple minority stress: The LGBT people of Color Microaggressions Scale. *Cultural Diversity & Ethnic Minority Psychology, 17*(2), 163–174. https://doi.org/10.1037/a0023244

Bennett, K. (1992). Feminist bisexuality: A both/and option for an either/or world. In E. R. Weise (Ed.), *Close to Home: Bisexuality and Feminism* (pp. 205–231). Seattle, WA: The Seal Press.

Bitterman, A., & Hess, D. B. (2020). Understanding generation gaps in LGBTQ+ communities: Perspectives about gay neighborhoods among heteronormative and homonormative generational cohorts. *The Life and Afterlife of Gay Neighborhoods: Renaissance and Resurgence*, 307–338. https://doi.org/10.1007/978-3-030-66073-4_14

Boppana, S., & Gross, A. M. (2019). The impact of religiosity on the psychological well-being of LGBT Christians. *Journal of Gay & Lesbian Mental Health, 23*(4), 412–426. http://doi.org/10.1080/19359705.2019.1645072

Buss, D. M. (1985). Human mate selection: Opposites are sometimes said to attract, but in fact we are likely to marry someone who is similar to us in almost every variable. *American Scientist, 73*(1), 47–51.

Eyre, S. L., Milbrath, C., & Peacock, B. (2007). Romantic relationships trajectories of African American gay/bisexual adolescents. *Journal of Adolescent Research, 22*(2), 107–131. http://doi.org/10.1177/0895904805298417

Festinger, L. (1962). Cognitive dissonance. *Scientific American, 207*(4), 93–107. http://doi.org/10.1038/scientificamerican1062-93

Floyd, F. J., & Stein, T. S. (2002). Sexual orientation identity formation among gay, lesbian, and bisexual youths: Multiple patterns of milestone experiences. *Journal of Research on Adolescence, 12*(2), 167–191. https://doi.org/10.1111/1532-7795.00030

Gaztambide, D. J. (2012). Addressing cultural impasses with rupture resolution strategies: A proposal and recommendations. *Professional Psychology: Research and Practice, 43*(3), 183–189. http://doi.org/10.1037/a0026911

Howden, D. (2011). Sistani renounces fatwa on gays. *The Independent*. Retrieved from www.independent.co.uk/news/world/middle-east/sistani-renounces-fatwa-on-gays-478396.html

Kim, H., Prouty, A. M., & Roberson, P. N. E. (2012). Narrative therapy with intercultural couples: A case study. *Journal of Family Psychotherapy, 23*(4), 273–286.

Kimmel, M. (2003). Adolescent masculinity, homophobia, and violence: Random school shootings, 1982–2001. *American Behavioral Scientist, 46*, 1439–1458.

Kinsey, A. C., Pomeroy, W. B., & Martin, C. E. (1948). *Sexual Behavior of the Human Male*. Philadelphia, PA: W.B. Saunders.

Kugle, S. S. al-Haqq. (2010). *Homosexuality in Islam: Critical Reflection on Gay, Lesbian, and Transgender Muslims.* Oxford: Oneworld.

Kumaraswamy, N. (2007). Psychotherapy in Brunei Darussalam. *Journal of Clinical Psychology: In Session, 63*, 735–744. http://doi.org/10.1002/jclp.20388

MacDonald, A. P. (1981). Bisexuality: Some comments on research and theory. *Journal of Homosexuality, 6*, 21–35.

Marsella, A. J. (2009). Some reflections on potential abuses of psychology's knowledge and practices. *Psychological Studies, 54*, 23–27. http://doi.org/10.1007/s12646-009-0003-8

Martin, D. J., Garske, J. P., & Davis, M. K. (2000). Relation of the therapeutic alliance with outcome and other variables: A meta-analytic review. *Journal of Consulting and Clinical Psychology, 68*(3), 438–450. http://doi.org/10.1037/0022-006X.68.3.438

McConnell, E. A., Janulis, P., Phillips, G., Truong, R., & Birkett, M. (2018). Multiple minority stress and LGBT community resilience among sexual minority men. *Psychology of Sexual Orientation and Gender Diversity, 5*(1), 1–12. https://doi.org/10.1037/sgd0000265

Meyer, I. H. (1995). Minority stress and mental health in gay men. *Journal of Health and Social Behavior, 36*, 38–56.

Mulick, P. S. (1999). *The Biphobia Scale: Development and Validation.* Masters Theses, https://scholarworks.wmich.edu/masters_theses/4124

Nardi, D., Waite, R., & Killian, P. (2012). Establishing standards for culturally competent mental health care. *Journal of Psychosocial Nursing and Mental Health Services, 50*(7), 3–5. http://doi.org/10.3928/02793695-20120608-01

Ong, C., Tan, R., Le, D., Tan, A., Tyler, A., Tan, C., Kwok, C., Banergee, S., & Wong, M. (2021). Association between sexual orientation acceptance and suicidal ideation, substance use, and internalised homophobia amongst the pink carpet Y cohort study of young gay, bisexual, and queer men in Singapore. *BMC Public Health, 21*, 971. https://doi.org/10.1186/s12889-021-10992-6

Patterson, G. E., Ward, D. B., & Brown, T. B. (2013). Relationship scripts: How young women develop and maintain same-sex romantic relationships. *Journal of GLBT Family Studies, 9*(2), 179–201. http://doi.org/10.1080/1550428X.2013.765263

Safran, J. D., Muran, J. C., & Eubanks-Carter, C. (2011). Repairing alliance ruptures. *Psychotherapy, 48*(1), 80–87. http://doi.org/10.1037/a0022140

Santini, Z. I., Koyanagi, A., Tyrovolas, S., & Haro, J. M. (2015). The association of relationship quality and social networks with depression, anxiety, and suicidal ideation among older married adults: Findings from a cross-sectional analysis of the Irish Longitudinal Study on aging. *Journal of Affective Disorders, 179*, 134–141. http://doi.org/10.1016/j.jad.2015.03.015

Storms, M. D. (1980). Theories of sexual orientation. *Journal of Personality and Social Psychology, 38*, 783–792.

Thies, K. E., Starks, T. J., Denmark, F. L., & Rosenthal, L. (2016). Internalized homonegativity and relationship quality in same-sex romantic couples: A test of mental health mechanisms and gender as a moderator. *Psychology of Sexual Orientation and Gender Diversity, 3*(3), 325–335. https://doi.org/10.1037/sgd0000183

Young, J. E., Klosko, J. S., & Weishaar, M. E. (2003). *Schema Therapy: A Practitioner's Guide.* New York: Guilford Press. ISBN 9781593853723. OCLC 51053419.

Zeidner, M., & Zevulun, A. (2017). Mental health and coping patterns in Jewish Gay Men in Israel: The role of dual identity conflict, religious identity, and partnership status. *Journal of Homosexuality, 65*(7), 947–968. http://doi.org/10.1080/00918369.2017.1364941

Chapter 10

Chronic health issues, disability and Queer people

Dr Alex Iantaffi

Introduction

Chronic health and disability are issues rarely discussed within both queer and therapeutic communities. This is not surprising given that *ableism*, which is the ideology that assumes that abled bodies are the standard and that indicates the systemic oppression of disabled people on a societal level, is pervasive within both contexts (Olkin et al., 2019). In addition to ableism, *sanism* is also ubiquitous within both communities, which is a system of systemic oppression of and discrimination against people who are considered to be "mad" or "mentally ill" according to current historical, sociocultural standards. Sanism is deeply rooted within Western psychological frameworks, which locate any mental health issues within the individual psyche rather than viewing those as manifestations of systemic issues (Leblanc & Kinsella, 2016).

When addressing chronic health issues and disabilities, we often tend to construe those as mainly physical rather than to consider all the ways in which our bodyminds (Price, 2015) exist. In fact, the term "bodymind" itself was coined to challenge the false dichotomy between our bodies and minds and highlight that we are integrated beings with bodies and minds that function in relation with one another. In this chapter, I will try to be as inclusive as possible of a broad range of chronic health and disability issues and to address how these might be intersecting with queer identities and experiences in particular. As well as discussing the construct of health and why it matters to include chronic health and disability issues in this volume on queer relationality, I will provide an overview of the various models of disability, from the medical model to the social model and some of the critiques this received by mostly feminist disabled scholars, to the framework of disability justice, which I utilize to illustrate the clinical vignettes included here before some final key points.

Chronic health or disability?

You might have noticed that, so far, I have used both *chronic health* and *disability* and might be asking yourselves why not pick one or the other. The decision to use both is to honour the fact that many people who experience chronic health issues

DOI: 10.4324/9781003260561-11

might not identify as disabled, often due to the pervasive influence of ableism and sanism, but also due to many people not being sure of where the line might lie between chronic health issues and disability if indeed there is a line. Just as some queer people might feel not "queer enough" and some trans people not "trans enough", some people with chronic health issues also feel "not disabled enough". This also points out the issue of binary thinking being problematic in many ways, including the ways in which we construe health and bodyminds (Barker & Iantaffi, 2019) as well as genders and sexualities.

What then can a definition of chronic health issues be? Within a medical model, a chronic health condition is one that continues or re-occurs over a period of time. Three months is sometimes used as the demarcation to indicate that conditions that last beyond this period of time are chronic (Bernell & Howard, 2016). Some chronic health issues are clear to both medical providers and the general public, such as diabetes or asthma, whereas others might be less known and might go undiagnosed for long periods of time. The definition of disability seems more dependent on the model adopted, as I will discuss in the next section. On a legal level, each country might, or might not, have a definition that is clearly highlighted in legislative acts, such as, for example, the Disability Discrimination Act 1995 in the UK or the Provisions on Assistance Benefiting Persons with Serious Disabilities Who Are Deprived of Family Support (Law No. 112–2016) in Italy. Legislative definitions are often based on the ability to work and/or to "function" according to abled and capitalist standards and based on a mythology of independence versus a lived reality of interdependence.

You may begin to notice that definitions of chronic health and disability are rather dependent on the ideological frameworks within which we operate, even though, at first glance, concepts like health seem simple and familiar. This is not dissimilar from the ways in which we define genders or sexualities, which are also rooted within dominant ideological frameworks rather than being the fixed entities that dominant discourse would have us believe. Before transitioning to briefly discussing why it matters to address issues of chronic health and disability, and before discussing the various models of disability, I want to add a note on why I am not using people-first language – such as people with disabilities – in this chapter. Although no community is homogeneous and individual people have a range of preferences, a majority of disabled people prefer to not use person-first language (Dunn & Andrews, 2015; Gernsbacher, 2017). Using the term "disabled people", for many, highlights that societal norms are the disabling factors, emphasizing the systemic instead of locating disability as individual "illness" (Ferrigon & Tucker, 2019). In this chapter, and in my writing in general, I want to emphasize the systemic as well, hence the use of disabled people, which I also use in my personal life as a disabled person. Consistent with this framework, I will use the term abled for people who are not disabled, as it has often been used by disability activists to emphasize how, if people are not disabled, they are implicitly enabled by current sociocultural, legal, educational and architectural norms.

Regardless of language used, why does it matter to address chronic health issues and disability in a volume on working with queer people in relationships?

It is estimated that, globally, 15% of people are disabled; that is a total of over a billion people (World Health Organization, 2011). Although these numbers are about a decade old now, they are still more up-to-date than the previously estimated 10% of the global population from the 1970s. Within Europe, the European Union recognized not only the importance of current numbers but also the ongoing impact of the COVID-19 pandemic and the possible impact on the number of disabled people, due to complications and Long Covid. This has led to a new Strategy for the Rights of Persons with Disabilities 2021–2030 (European Commission, 2021) to address existing and potentially growing inequalities.

We could say that disabled people, and those with chronic health issues, are one of the largest, if not the largest, minoritised population across the globe, yet our existence, issues, and experiences are often erased, ignored, or overlooked. This is no different within the field of relationship therapy within which resources for disabled trans and queer people are often non-existent or are created within an ableist framework by abled people rather than by disabled queer and trans people ourselves. Before moving on to discussing the intersection of queerness and disability, though, I want to introduce the various theoretical lenses through which we can view this.

Models of disability

The theoretical lens we adopt is highly influential on how we view ourselves, others and the world around us. This is also true when addressing the topic of this chapter. I have already mentioned how ableism and sanism are ubiquitous within dominant discourse. For example, disabled people are often depicted as innocent angels (Santos & Santos, 2018) or villains in popular media (Leary, 2017), or lifted up as "brave and courageous", something that is usually referred to as "inspiration porn" by disabled people (Schalk, 2021). I will discuss how this impacts disabled people's sexualities later, but for now, let's take a look at some of the major lenses through which we can view disability and chronic health issues.

The medical model is probably the best known because it is all around us within dominant discourses in most Western countries, including the United Kingdom and the European Union. Within this model, disability is a chronic condition that can be assessed, quantified and addressed on an individual level. We are disabled, or chronically ill, if our bodyminds do not function according to medical standards of functioning, which is within a clinical taxonomy (Marks, 1997). You might have noticed, for example, that I did not use terms such as physically, cognitively or psychiatrically disabled. However, those are categories often used within clinical taxonomy. They can also be found within education systems, which are also steeped in the medical model of disability. Within this model, chronic health and disability are a deficit indicating that something is not working as it "should". Legislation is often founded on the clinical model as it is not only quantifiable but also compatible with legal taxonomies.

Within this model, we find words such as "impairment", "special needs", "accommodations", and theories such as "learned helplessness". The idea is that there is a deviation from abled norms, which are viewed as preferable and not needing to be accommodated. In fact, there are usually no accommodations needed for abled people because the norms inherently accommodate them. For example, it is fairly common for most people to have a cell phone nowadays. However, devices used for augmentative and/or assisted communication (AAC), that is communication boards, head pointers, speech synthesizers and so on, are expensive, not easily available and construed as exceptional and, at times, as engendering dependence for those who use them. Yet, despite most people's dependence on cell phones, we do not worry that abled people will become so dependent on their phones that they will no longer be able to communicate in ways that people find acceptable. This is because cell phone use has been normalized within dominant culture, whereas the use of other communication aids is viewed as different and exceptional.

Within the medical model, diagnosis is foundational and necessary to access support services and devices, as well as care. Most providers, including psychologists and other mental health providers, are trained within this framework. If some of the terms used here, such as "impairment" or "special needs", seem more familiar to you, it is because they are likely consistent with the theoretical framework within which you were trained as a mental health provider.

In the mid-1970s, the disability movement started to gain momentum, and in 1976, *The Fundamental Principles of Disability* was published in London, UK, by the Union of the Physically Impaired Against Segregation, stating that "in our view, it is a society that disables physically impaired people. Disability is something imposed on top of our impairments by the way we are unnecessarily isolated and excluded from full participation in society" (UPIAS, 1976, p. 14). The social model of disability is born. Within this model, we are disabled, not due to failure(s) of our bodyminds, but rather those of society. For example, if a wheelchair user cannot enter a building, it is due to stairs being standard and a lack of ramps and/or appropriate elevators. If a Deaf person cannot attend a theatre performance, it is not because of a "hearing impairment" but rather due to the lack of open captioning and/or sign language interpreters.

This model has been used within several social justice communities for the past thirty years and it is, at times, still put forward as the alternative to a medical model when discussing disability (Oliver, 2013). However, several critiques regarding this model came from disabled feminist scholars and activists who pointed out that this model swung so far opposite from the medical model that it ended up erasing and ignoring the embodied experiences of many disabled people. In the 1990s, feminist disabled activists and writers, such as Liz Crow (1992), Sally French (1993) and Jenny Morris (1991), among others, highlighted that, while placing emphasis on systemic issues on a societal level is vital, we can do so without denying the material existence and experiences of the body. For example, we do not need to deny that many of us experience pain, or have sensory limitations, such as poor vision, that impact the ways in which we interact with ourselves, others and the world around us. As feminists, they advocated for an approach to disability that is both social and personal, knowing that the personal is indeed political.

Around the same time, feminist disabled scholars Potts and Price (1995) argued, in the US, that to deny the materiality of academic production, that is the demands that academic labour places on our bodyminds, is most impactful on disabled women, given that erasure of the body usually serves patriarchal systems best. It is, in fact, no accident that the social model of disability emerges from the scholarship of cisgender white men, who do not seem to be as aware of, or impacted by, the material labour of academia. It is within these feminist critiques of the social model of disability that we can appreciate how disability and/or chronic health issues cannot be considered as separate from a systemic analysis of power and privilege that also includes gender, sexuality, class and race.

It is also at the intersection of gender, queer studies and disability studies that crip theory emerges (McRuer, 2006). This can be viewed, in simplistic terms, as the combination of queer studies with disability studies, and it is often categorized as a sub-set of the larger field of disability studies. Crip theory is intersectional as it pays attention to issues of race, gender and class as well as disability through a systemic analysis of power. While I will not address this here, as it is beyond the scope of this chapter, it is worth mentioning its existence, and that the theoretical field of crip studies has also engendered both supporters and critics. Around the same time that this field begins to establish itself, a new framework, Disability Justice, emerges within the United States, led by people of colour, as well as trans and queer activists.

Disability Justice, as a term, is first used in the early 2000s in a conversation amongst queer disabled women of colour, including Patty Berne, Mia Mingus and Stacey Milbern. They soon began collaborating with other trans and queer disabled activists, such as Eli Clare, Leroy Moore and Sebastian Margaret (Berne, 2015; Berne et al., 2018), and from these collaborations the Disability Justice Collective was born. Within this framework, every bodymind is whole, while recognizing that systems of power and oppression target some of us as candidates for ongoing eugenic practices, that is, the ideology that humans can be improved by selecting "desirable" traits for reproduction and eliminating those who are less "desirable".

This is an intersectional framework in that it adopts a systemic analysis of power, including recognizing how we cannot address ableism and sanism without addressing colonialism, neo-Imperialism, capitalism, misogyny, white supremacy, anti-Blackness, transphobia and queerphobia. Those legacies are just as intertwined as our liberation is, and they impact those who are historically and systematically minoritised, such as not only disabled people but also immigrants, working-class people, Black and Brown and other racialized people, trans, non-binary, gender-expansive and queer people (Piepzna-Samarasinha, 2018).

While disability justice is a living framework in progress, ten principles have been identified by its founders (Berne et al., 2018, Sins Invalid, 2015):

- Intersectionality.
- Leadership of those most impacted.
- Anti-capitalist politic.
- Commitment to cross-movement organizing.
- Recognizing wholeness.
- Sustainability.
- Commitment to cross-disability solidarity.
- Interdependence.
- Collective access.
- Collective liberation.

These principles will inform the clinical vignettes presented later in this chapter, but for now, let's turn to consider the intersection of disability and queerness in a little more depth.

Disabled and queer

Queer people, especially non-white queer and trans people, have often built inter-movement solidarity, as depicted, for example, in *Pride*, a British movie based on a true story in which some queer activists organize to raise funds for the families of striking miners, for what would become the "Lesbians and Gays Support Miners" campaign in the mid-1980s. Like other minoritised communities, many of us have long understood how our liberation is indeed linked to one another.

Disabled queer people have often needed to advocate for access within queer and trans spaces, while also advocating for gender and sexual equality within some disabled spaces. More often than not, though, disabled people have been invisible within queer movements, especially those led by cisgender white people campaigning for assimilation into a capitalist, homonormative ideal, rather than for the liberation of all bodyminds that have been considered "deviant" and "unworthy" within dominant discourses. Even though, from the 1980s onwards, our queer communities have experienced higher numbers of people living with HIV, compared to heterosexual people, we seem to have separated those experiences from those of our fellow queers disabled by conditions other than, or as well as, HIV.

As well as experiencing invisibility and, at times, erasure within queer communities, disabled queer people experience also what disabled heterosexual people experience within the broader community, especially in relation to sexuality, that is infantilisation and desexualisation (Haller & Zhang, 2014). Infantilisation refers to the phenomenon of abled people construing disabled people as innocent and ignorant children, rather than granting them autonomy and agency. Most disabled and chronically ill people have experienced this, especially if their disabilities and/or chronic health issues are visible to others, through the use of mobility aids, for example. This can include abled people talking down to disabled people and talking to people who they read as abled even when they should be addressing the disabled person present, such as when taking their order at a restaurant. Sometimes abled people not only talk down to disabled people, but even babble as if they were talking to a baby, other times they might grab our assistive devices, such as wheelchairs, walkers or canes, without asking for consent, and might even get angry and aggressive when this is pointed out to them.

Infantilisation impacts queer and trans people in specific ways as well. Disabled people already have less access to sex education than our abled peers, for example, because of being thought of as children who need to be protected from "adult topics", such as sex (Fiduccia, 2000). This means that trans and queer disabled youth often have little to no access to information, and yet, as disabled youth, they are more likely to experience sexual abuse by caregivers, educators and peers, especially in residential settings, including schools (Paul & Cawson, 2002; Sullivan & Knutson, 2000). Given that most sexual education does not include gender, sexual and relational diversity, the paucity of sex education for disabled young people impacts trans and queer youth even more than their heterosexual peers. Even young adults, or adults, might be considered "unable" to claim a trans and/or queer identity as valid due to being presumed incompetent by able people around them, such as family members, educators, caregivers, co-workers and healthcare providers. This benevolent yet dangerous "protection" not only endangers disabled trans and queer people but also creates obstacles when trying to access care and support around having experienced sexual violence and abuse (Brown, 2017).

In addition to infantilisation, as stated earlier, disabled people also experience desexualisation. I am purposefully using desexualisation, rather than asexualisation, as the latter erases and renders invisible disabled asexual and/or aromantic people who do, in fact, exist. Whatever our sexual, relational or gender identities, many disabled people are considered to be either not sexual, or to have "chosen" a trans, queer or non-monogamous identity because of our disability. The experience of having gender, sexual and/or relational identities other than cisgender, heterosexual and monogamous invalidated by abled people around us is not uncommon for many disabled people. Those identities as queer, or kinky, are considered to be stemming from our "inability" to conform to cis-heteronormative standards of sex, depriving us, once more, of legitimacy and agency. Even when disabled people are hypersexualised, such as when amputees are fetishised (try to Google amputees and devotees, for example), that could be considered a form of desexualisation as it divests us of common humanity. Disabled trans feminine people, especially those who are racialized as not white, in particular, experience these types of desexualisation, including hypersexualisation and vilification, in ways that are specific to the intersection of trans misogyny and racism (Arnold & Bonython, 2021; Bolivar, 2018; Holmes, 2016).

The desexualisation of disabled people rests on the tenet that we are somehow "unfuckable" and lacking in erotic capital within ableist, patriarchal, colonial, classist and racist paradigms. Although, within these paradigms, we might, at times, have erotic capital as, usually non-consensual, fetishes (Gowland, 2002). Once again, trans people, Black, Brown and other racialised people, immigrants, and lower-class people are especially impacted due to also being non-consensually exoticised and hypersexualised in specific ways. We can also notice the absence of disabled people as sex workers, rather than just consumers of sex work, as yet another example of erasure through desexualisation. We cannot be legitimate sexual subjects, but we can, at times, be sexual objects, either as fetishes or consumers. This is particularly impactful for those of us who are also queer and, as such, are already not granted full sexual citizenship because of our sexualities. Those of us who are disabled and non-monogamous also face similar issues (Iantaffi, 2022). Now that we have considered how disability and chronic health issues impact the sexualities of queer people, let's consider some clinical examples. Please note that all the following clinical examples are fictional vignettes and not stories of actual therapy clients.

Working therapeutically with trans and queer disabled people

There is very little literature on disability, chronic health issues and sexuality, especially within the field of mental health (Iantaffi & Mize, 2015; Iantaffi, 2022). What little is available is often rooted within a medical model. I hope that the examples in this section, and the accompanying connections drawn with some of the disability justice principles, might offer you a new, or at least affirming, perspective.

Vignette 1

Gina has lived in the UK for about three years. She is a white, Spanish graduate student pursuing a PhD in Clinical Psychology. Gina has been living with myalgic encephalomyelitis (ME), most commonly referred to as chronic fatigue syndrome (CFS), for the past year. She has recently married her partner, Joy, a white, English woman who is ten years older than Gina is, but their wedding day was clouded by the absence of Joy's parents, who don't approve of their relationship and consider Gina to be "lazy" and "taking advantage" of their daughter. Gina and Joy have come to therapy to address Gina's feelings towards Joy's family, given that Joy keeps seeing them even though Gina is not welcome at Joy's parents' home.

Take a pause to consider this scenario. . . . I encourage you to record your thoughts in some way, whether by writing them down, or dictating yourself a voice memo as you will be asked to revisit them later.

- When you receive this referral, what do you notice?
- What are you curious about and want to find out more about?
- What are your hypotheses about this case based on the information you have?
- What information do you want to prioritise collecting?
- How does your positionality inform all of the above?
- Where does your positionality converge, and where does it diverge from those of Gina and Joy?
- What theoretical approaches, skills and interventions do you think might be most helpful with this case?
- If you were to consider this case through the lens of the principle of "leadership of those most impacted", would anything change? Who is most impacted in this scenario, not just on a personal level, but on a systemic level? Why? How might this principle impact the way you approach this couple?
- If you were to consider this case through the lens of "sustainability", would anything you have already considered change? What does sustainability mean for Gina and Joy in their life as a couple?
- How might the principle of sustainability impact your therapeutic relationship with Gina and Joy? What factors do you imagine might hinder or nurture sustainability in the therapeutic relationship between you and this couple?

Now take a moment to consider whether any of your thoughts and considerations might change when you find out, during the course of your therapeutic relationship, that Gina comes from a financially well-off, solidly middle-class, and supportive family, whereas Joy comes from a working-class family and has never experienced financial security before meeting Gina. If anything changes, why? If not, why not? How is this information relevant, or not, when considering the principles of "leadership of those most impacted" and of "sustainability"?

Do any of your thoughts and considerations so far change when you find out that they have started to talk about having children together in a year or two? If so, how do they change and why? If not, why not? Finally, what attitudes, values, biases and beliefs have you noticed as you considered this clinical scenario. Please try to notice these with as much curiosity, honesty and non-judgement as you can muster at this moment.

Vignette 2

Chris, Kevin and Roger are considering moving in together. Kevin and Roger have been together for just over ten years, and their relationship has been non-monogamous throughout. Although they both dated during these ten years, this is the first time that they are considering living with one of their partners. Chris has been dating Roger for just over a year and has become close friends with Kevin during this time. Kevin has recently been diagnosed with Dissociative Identity Disorder (DID), which was both overwhelming and a relief for them as well as for Roger. Previously, neither of them had been able to make sense of some intense mood shifts between them, as well as of inconsistent patterns of sexual desire and behaviours. Roger is worried that Chris moving in with them might be destabilising for Kevin right now. He is also not sure how Chris might react to Kevin during times when they can be rather detached, especially as she has a history of childhood trauma, is neurodivergent, and has openly shared that she has an anxious attachment style, which has created issues in some of her past relationships. They have come to see you to discuss all this in therapy before deciding how to move forward.

Once again, take your time to take in this scenario. . . . Please remember to record your thoughts, questions and wonderings in some way. This time I am going to invite you to reflect on this scenario through the disability justice principles of "recognising wholeness" and "commitment to cross-disability solidarity".

- Would you accept working with these clients or not? If so, why, and if not, why not?
- Would your decision to work with them change based on their positionalities, and if so, why? If not, why not?
- What do you imagine the goal of therapy to be in this scenario?
- How would you address discussions of potentially competing needs within the relationships in this system, as well as within a potential combined household?
- How might the principles of recognising wholeness and commitment to cross-disability solidarity guide your therapeutic work in this case?
- How might sanism show up in your therapeutic encounters with this relationship configuration?
- What assumptions, values, biases and beliefs do you notice as you consider this case? Again with as much curiosity and non-judgement as you are able at this moment.
- How does your positionality inform the way you approach each of these clients, their relationships with one another, and the relational system as a whole?
- What other information do you need to address this scenario?
- What positionalities do you imagine Chris, Kevin and Roger to have with regards to age, race, ethnicity, immigration status, gender, sexuality, class, level of education, socioeconomic level and religion? If you change the positionalities you imagine them to have, how does that change your therapeutic approach, if at all, and why?

Once again, take your thoughts and reflections in as information to help you evaluate your own attitudes, values, beliefs and biases, and to assess what support you might need, if any, to work in an affirming and effective way with a scenario like the one offered here.

Vignette 3

Bilan is a Somali-Italian, Black trans woman in her mid-30s. She works as a high school teacher, is a practising Muslim, and is close to her parents and brother who live in the same city. She divorced shortly before sharing her gender with people in her life, including at work, and has been single for the past five years. Bilan would like to start dating again but is nervous about a number of issues. She has experienced transphobia, racism and Islamophobia the few times she has gone down to a bar or club with some of her close friends. Bilan is worried about her safety if she uses an app or website for online dating, which seems to be how most of her friends date nowadays. She has never dated as her first marriage was arranged and feels both old and naive. One of her additional concerns is that she is a wheelchair user, which, she feels, could make her more vulnerable if she goes out on a date by herself. She has come to you for support and advice.

Take a pause to consider this scenario, this time through the lens of the principles of "intersectionality" and "collective liberation".

- What are the first thoughts and reactions you notice, again, with as much honesty, curiosity and non-judgement as you are able at this moment? What are your second thoughts and reactions after the first ones? Are they similar or different? What informs both your first thoughts and reactions and your second thoughts and reactions?
- What do you imagine your role as a therapist to be in this therapeutic scenario? What theoretical framework and practices inform what you imagine your role as a therapist to be in this case?
- When you consider this vignette through the lens of intersectionality, what aspects seem more prominent or time-sensitive to address if any?
- What are the assumptions that Bilan is making in this situation? Are your assumptions about her situation similar or different from the ones you imagine her to have?
- What therapeutic concepts might be useful when you consider this case and why?
- What theory of change do you think might be effective in working with Bilan?
- Are there interventions that you would use when working with this client? If so, what are the assumptions underpinning your choice of interventions?
- Do you imagine the therapeutic goal to remain the same or to change through the course of your work with Bilan? If so, what might influence the change of therapeutic goal(s) in this situation, and why?
- In every therapeutic relationship, we risk harming our clients if we are not intentional, thoughtful and ethical. What do you think you need to particularly pay attention to in this case to avoid potential harm? If harm occurs,

what kind of harm do you imagine it might be? Would repair be possible if Bilan was available and willing to engage in this? If so, what could a repair process be like?

- How can the principle of collective liberation be applied to this scenario? How could this guide your therapeutic approach in working with Bilan?

Just as you have done previously, take a moment to notice what information might be valuable for you, as a clinician, after working with this vignette. What have you learned? Did anything surprise you? If so, what?

After reflecting on all three vignettes, and what you noticed from your responses to the prompts offered, are there things you would want to change in your practice? If so, what and why? If not, what are things that you appreciate and feel affirmed around, within your clinical practice, in relation to queerness, relationships and disability? If you can, take time to notice and record not just your thoughts but also your feelings, somatic reactions such as sensations in your body, images, impulses and narratives that might emerge after reading this chapter and engaging with the clinical vignettes offered.

Final key points for consideration and reflection

- What is the difference between chronic health issues and disability, if any? If there is a difference, where does it stem from?
- Does the meaning of health vary according to the theoretical lens adopted? If so, what is your lens and what does "health" mean to you and within your practice?
- When considering the models of disability presented in this chapter (medical, social, feminist and disability justice), which ones feel familiar and which ones do not? Are any of the models uncomfortable, and if so, can you identify why? Do any of the models fit better than others with your existing worldviews? If so, which one(s) and why?
- Do the ten principles of disability justice offer something of value to your clinical practice? If so, what is it and why? How can applying them change, or further affirm, the way you work?
- What are all the ways in which disability, gender, queerness and relationships intersect with one another in your life and within your clinical practice? How do they inform your positionality, and the positionalities of your colleagues, clients and supervisees (if you are a supervisor)?
- Are there clients you would refer, or not, or work differently with after engaging with this chapter? Why?
- Which reflective practices, both individual and relational, might you adopt, develop and/or nurture after reading this chapter?
- How would you nurture your bodymind as a clinician, if you were to adopt the ten principles of disability justice as guides in your work?

References

Arnold, B. B., & Bonython, W. (2021). Some are more equal than others? Dignity, difference and vilification. *Griffith Journal of Law & Human Dignity, 8*(2).

Barker, M. J., & Iantaffi, A. (2019). *Life Isn't Binary*. London: Jessica Kingsley Publishers.

Berne, P. (2015). *Disability Justice – A Working Draft*. San Francisco: Sins Invalid.

Berne, P., Morales, A. L., Langstaff, D., & Invalid, S. (2018). Ten principles of disability justice. *WSQ: Women's Studies Quarterly, 46*(1), 227–230.

Bernell, S., & Howard, S. W. (2016). Use your words carefully: What is a chronic disease? *Frontiers in Public Health, 4*, 159.

Bolivar, A. (2018). We are a fantasia: Violence, belonging, and potentiality in transgender Latina sexual economies. *Arts & Sciences Electronic Theses and Dissertations, 1512*. Retrieved from https://openscholarship.wustl.edu/art_sci_etds/1512

Brown, L. X. (2017). Ableist shame and disruptive bodies: Survivorship at the intersection of queer, trans, and disabled existence. In *Religion, Disability, and Interpersonal Violence* (pp. 163–178). Cham: Springer.

Crow, L. (1992). Renewing the social model of disability. *Roaring Girl Productions* [online]. Retrieved August 30, 2022, from www.roaring-girl.com/work/renewing-the-social-model-of-disability/

Dunn, D. S., & Andrews, E. E. (2015). Person-first and identity-first language: Developing psychologists' cultural competence using disability language. *American Psychologist, 70*(3), 255.

European Commission. (2021). *Strategy for Rights of Persons with Disabilities 2021–2030*. Retrieved September 14, 2021, from https://ec.europa.eu/commission/presscorner/api/files/document/print/en/qanda_21_813/QAN DA_21_813_EN.pdf

Ferrigon, P., & Tucker, K. (2019). Person-first language vs. Identity-first language: An examination of the gains and drawbacks of Disability Language in society. *Journal of Teaching Disability Studies*. Retrieved from https://jtds.commons.gc.cuny.edu/person-first-language-vs-identity-first-language-an-examination-of-the-gains-and-drawbacks-of-disability-language-in-society/

Fiduccia, B. W. (2000). Current issues in sexuality and the disability movement. *Sexuality and Disability, 18*(3), 167–174.

French, S. (1993). Disability, impairment or something in between? In J. Swain, V. Finkelstein, S. French, & M. Oliver (Eds.), *Disabling Barriers – Enabling Environments* (pp. 17–25). Maidenhead, UK: Sage Publications, Inc; Open University Press.

Gernsbacher, M. A., (2017). Editorial perspective: The use of person first language in scholarly writing may accentuate stigma. *Journal of Child Psychology and Psychiatry, 58*(7), 859–861.

Gowland, R. (2002). Freak fucker: Stereotypical representations of sexuality in British disability art. *Disability Studies Quarterly, 22*(4).

Haller, B., & Zhang, L. (2014). Stigma or empowerment? What do disabled people say about their representation in news and entertainment media? *Review of Disability Studies: An International Journal, 9*(4).

Holmes, C. M. (2016). The colonial roots of the racial fetishization of black women. *Black & Gold, 2*(1).

Iantaffi, A. (2022). Disability & CNM relationships. In T. Burnes & M. Vaughan (Eds.), *Handbook of CNM-Affirming Clinical Practice*. Lanham, MD: Rowman & Littlefield Publishers.

Iantaffi, A., & Mize, S. (2015). Disability. In *The Palgrave Handbook of the Psychology of Sexuality and Gender* (pp. 408–426). London: Palgrave Macmillan.

Leary, A. (2017). How disfigured villains like wonder woman's Dr. Poison Perpetuate Stigma. *Teen Vogue*, 5.

Leblanc, S., & Kinsella, E. A. (2016). Toward epistemic justice: A critically reflexive examination of 'sanism and implications for knowledge generation. *Studies in Social Justice*, *10*(1), 59–78.

Marks, D. (1997). Models of disability. *Disability and Rehabilitation*, *19*(3), 85–91.

McRuer, R. (2006). *Crip Theory: Cultural Signs of Queerness and Disability* (Vol. 9). New York: NYU Press.

Morris, J. (1991). *Pride Against Prejudice: Transforming Attitudes to Disability*. London: The Women's Press.

Oliver, M. (2013). The social model of disability: Thirty years on. *Disability & Society*, *28*(7), 1024–1026.

Olkin, R., Hayward, H. S., Abbene, M. S., & VanHeel, G. (2019). The experiences of microaggressions against women with visible and invisible disabilities. *Journal of Social Issues*, *75*(3), 757–785.

Paul, A., & Cawson, P. (2002). Safeguarding disabled children in residential settings: What we know and what we don't know. *Child Abuse Review: Journal of the British Association for the Study and Prevention of Child Abuse and Neglect*, *11*(5), 262–281.

Piepzna-Samarasinha, L. L. (2018). *Care Work: Dreaming Disability Justice*. Vancouver: Arsenal Pulp Press.

Potts, T., & Price, J. (1995). Out of the blood and spirit of our lives: The place of the body in academic feminism. *Feminist Academics. Creative Agents for Change*, 102–115.

Price, M. (2015). The bodymind problem and the possibilities of pain. *Hypatia*, *30*(1), 268–284.

Santos, A. C., & Santos, A. L. (2018). Yes, we fuck! Challenging the misfit sexual body through disabled women's narratives. *Sexualities*, *21*(3), 303–318.

Schalk, S. (2021). Black disability gone viral: A critical race approach to inspiration porn. *CLA Journal*, *64*(1), 100–120.

Sins Invalid. (2015). 10 principles of disability justice. *Sins Invalid Blog*. Retrieved January 15, 2022, from https://static1.squarespace.com/static/5bed3674f8370ad8c02efd9a/t/5f1f0783916d8a179c46126d/1595869064521/10_Principles_of_DJ-2ndEd.pdf

Sullivan, P. M., & Knutson, J. F. (2000). Maltreatment and disabilities: A population-based epidemiological study. *Child Abuse & Neglect*, *24*(10), 1257–1273.

UPIAS. (1976). *Fundamental Principles of Disability*. London: Union of the Physically Impaired Against Segregation.

World Health Organization and The World Bank. (2011). *World Report on Disability*. Geneva: World Health Organization. Retrieved September 14, 2021, from www.who.int/publications/i/item/9789241564182

The impact of antiretroviral therapies and PrEP on gay men

Guillermo Llorca

In 2006 I was discussing my stress levels with my GP:

> "And what do you do for a living?" she asked.
> "I work in a charity supporting LGBT people with mental health problems".
> "Have you ever had an HIV test?" was her immediate response.

I hadn't discussed nor disclosed my sexual orientation to my GP, and I wasn't talking about my sexual health or my sex practices. Nevertheless, when I mentioned "gay", the focus of my appointment shifted from my health issues to HIV (Human Immunodeficiency Virus). Gayness was and is attached to HIV. How was this link made? How has it affected gay men in their lives, and how is it changing with Antiretroviral Therapies (ART) and Pre-exposure Prophylaxis (PrEP), with the biomedicalisation of gay sex?

In the context of this chapter, I use the term "gay men" to include bisexual, queer, and other cis and trans men who have sex with men.

Since the beginning of the HIV and AIDS (Acquired Immune Deficiency Syndrome) epidemic in the early 1980s, gay men have been particularly affected by HIV and AIDS. In Western countries, AIDS was initially known as the "gay cancer", the "gay plague" and, formally, as Gay-Related Immune Deficiency (GRID) (Catalan et al., 2020; Florêncio, 2020), affecting and killing hundreds of thousands of gay men.

The HIV epidemic crisis began, coincidentally, when gay men had started enjoying the benefits of the gay liberation movement. For years, death, isolation, disease and health problems were intimately connected with gay men in the social imaginary. The HIV epidemic that initially impacted Sub-Saharan Africa seemed to have been created by a bigot, or by God, bigots would say, particularly affecting gay men, heroin addicts and people with haemophilia; the latter being, according to the Daily Express newspaper, the "AIDS innocents" (Crewe, 2018).

HIV, Gay men and the arse

Gay men are specially affected by HIV because of the prevalence of condomless anal sex in gay sex practices (in the past, promiscuity was often mentioned as a reason for this prevalence; Bolton, 1992).

DOI: 10.4324/9781003260561-12

If somebody with a detectable HIV viral load ejaculates inside during anal sex, the semen is absorbed directly into the bloodstream of the person being penetrated. Penetrating anally somebody who has a detectable HIV viral load is also a risky practice because of the high concentration of HIV inside the anus, which can be absorbed by the glans of the penis during penetration.

According to the Collins English Dictionary (2018), masculine in British English means "possessing qualities or characteristics considered typical of or appropriate to a man; manly; unwomanly". In *Por el culo. Políticas anales* [Up the Arse. Anal Politics], Carrascosa and Sáez (2011) write [my translation from Spanish]:

> if masculinity is not in the genitals (there are masculine cis women, and there are trans men who are men without "masculine" genitals), nor in hormones . . . where is it? Masculinity is in the arse, more specific, in its impenetrability. Of course, this is true only within the heterocentric and male chauvinistic regime.

According to Carrascosa and Sáez (2011), masculinity is defined by men's arses. Men penetrate and women are penetrated; men emit opinions and women receive opinions. A man is impenetrable (not mouth nor anus). In the Western dualism right/left, superior/inferior, man/woman, good/bad, anal sex between men would challenge and pervert this dualism. Men who enjoy being penetrated would question the meaning of masculinity.

The perception of anal intercourse as a disgusting practice is intimately connected to homonegativity (Morrison et al., 2019). The "arse" is dirty and abject. Gay men with behaviours considered as non-gender conforming, such as having "female personality" or adopting a receptive sexual role (being bottom), encounter more negative reactions and disgust than other gay men (Caswell & Sackett-Fox, 2018). While many gay men don't enjoy anal penetration, the stereotype would explain the link between patriarchy and homophobia with HIV related stigma.

Trauma

The experience of growing up and living in a heteronormative society has longlasting consequences on gay men's health and well-being. According to the Minority Stress Model (Meyer, 2003), minority stigmatised groups experience excess of stress that is unique to them. This stress can be divided into the following:

1   External prejudice and violence.
2   Expectations of discrimination and prejudice resulting in chronic vigilance regarding own safety (changing, for example, attitudes, mannerisms, clothing or refraining from exhibiting any form of intimacy with partners in public).
3   Internalised homophobia (perceiving yourself from the negative point of view of the other).

4   Constantly assessing the safety of disclosing/concealing own sexual
     orientation.

Mainstream gay culture may exacerbate gay men's minority stress in what
Pachankis et al. (2020) refer to as "intraminority stress" within the gay community. According to their study, attractiveness, masculinity and wealth can be
considered indicators of status within the gay community. Whereby, those with
self-perceived lower status will experience higher levels of stress and exclusion
when rejected by other gay men, particularly of higher status. Within the gay community, other elements associated with excess of stress and poor mental health
symptoms are the focus on sex and competition as well as exclusion of diversity.
Ultimately, it would seem gay communities mirror, and in some respects enhance,
the patriarchy, homonegativity and consumerism of mainstream society.

Trauma is a psychophysical response to an event a person finds highly stressful
(Rothschild, 2000). This could be any situation in which the individual perceives
their life or body integrity is at risk. It could involve specific incidents such as
sexual assault, an accident or a serious illness. It can also entail long-term events
such as neglected childhood, bullying, harassment or domestic violence. Lastly,
it could involve witnessing or hearing traumatic events of others. The definition
of trauma according to the DSM-5 (APA, 2013) focuses on the symptoms that a
highly distressful event can provoke. Moreover, Alessi et al. (2013) assert: "experiencing an event involving prejudice, regardless of severity, could cause PTSD
symptoms such as hypervigilance, fear, anxiety, and relationship problems"
(2013, p. 9). Considering that some of the homophobic and heterosexist prejudice
events that create an excess of stress and distress are repetitive and with different
levels of intensity, gay men may experience chronic and complex trauma-like
responses as a result.

During an initial consultation, a young gay man explained he wanted psychotherapy to help him remain in the closet, be able to marry a woman and find a way
to be happy living a straight life. He was short of requesting conversion therapy.
As a psychotherapist with integrity, it wasn't ethically possible to agree to his
proposed treatment; he understood my decision and went to look for a different
therapist.

In addition to the trauma of homophobia, the overlapping HIV related stigma
has been experienced by people living with HIV and vicariously by gay men
regardless of their HIV status, including internalised HIV stigma. This is similar
to the homophobia experienced by HIV activists and HIV+ heterosexual men in
some countries. Since the beginning of the epidemic, the risk of death (physical
or social) has been related to same-sex desire and gay sexuality. This has made a
perfect trauma storm. Overlapping stigmas can multiply for gay men who are, for
example, trans, from ethnic minority groups or from marginalised social classes.

Among gay clients (and also colleagues and friends), there are numerous
instances of this association between their sexual orientation and HIV regardless
of their status (Figure 11.1). Peter, whose father asked him after his breakdown,

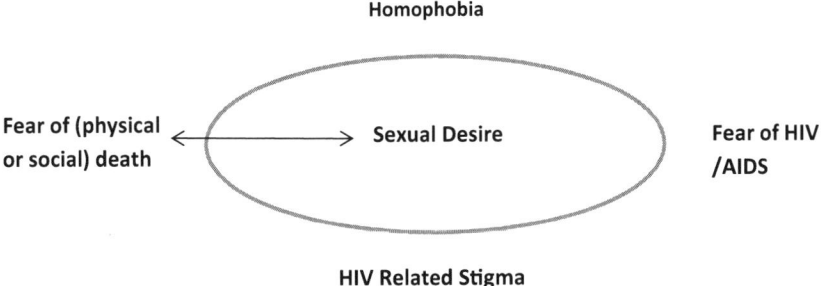

Homophobia

Fear of (physical or social) death ← → **Sexual Desire** → Fear of HIV /AIDS

HIV Related Stigma

Trauma in Gay Men

before ART and PrEP implementation

Figure 11.1 Trauma in gay men before ART and PrEP implementation.

"What's wrong? Did you catch AIDS?"; Paul, whose mother told him "I'm just worried you will get AIDS" when he came out to her; or Jon recounting his loneliness as a young teenager worrying about his first sexual encounters, his fear of HIV and having nobody to talk to about it.

ART

Since the introduction of ART in 1996, people with HIV on effective treatment maintain healthy lives. Their CD4 count remains high (meaning high immunity), and their viral load becomes undetectable. Therefore, HIV cannot progress into AIDS. This also means there isn't enough viral load in their bloodstream to be able to pass HIV to another person: "undetectable equals untransmittable". U = U was a campaign launched in 2016 by the Prevention Access Campaign, an organisation with the goal of ending the HIV epidemic as well as the HIV related stigma. This campaign has now been endorsed by a multitude of organisations around the world (Eisinger et al., 2019). U = U means ART works also as secondary HIV prevention: "Treatment as Prevention" (TasP). Most HIV transmissions happen during condomless penetrative sex when one is unaware of their HIV+ status. They believe they are "clean". Clean is a term used by many gay men when discussing HIV and other STIs. "Are you 'clean'? If you are 'clean', I'm happy to bareback". With the antonym of clean being dirty, living with HIV would imply "being dirty". Chemsex (crystal meth, GHB or mephedrone use during sex) is also an HIV high risk transmission activity (see Chapter 12 in *Erotically Queer*).

For ART to be effective, adherence to treatment is paramount. For years, adherence has been a complex matter; initially it required a serious commitment due to the numerous tablets to be taken throughout the day as well as their strong long-term side effects. ART has improved dramatically, particularly in wealthy countries, making adherence much easier. Nowadays, sometimes only a single-tablet regime is needed, and the new medication tends to have mild or milder side effects (single-tablet treatment availability may vary depending on the country). Adherence can still be complex due to mental health problems, trauma presentations and HIV stigma. Some individuals would experience their tablets as a daily reminder of their HIV related trauma, and they resort to, for example, forgetting to take their medication as a maladaptive coping mechanism, thus sabotaging their treatment and health. I recall a client somatising to the point of physically struggling to swallow their medication. Poor adherence to ART not only affects its effectiveness but also can mean the organism becomes resistant to that specific treatment. Nevertheless, ART has been successful thanks to the individuals' commitment to their medication adherence. Still, worldwide many people with HIV may not have access to ART.

Case I

Ramón is a middle-aged gay cis man who grew up in a small town in Argentina; the youngest of three siblings with emotionally distant parents. He lived in Buenos Aires for most of his adulthood. Ramón never came out to his family, "but they know. We just don't talk about these things". He had had two significant intimate relationships that, according to him, ended "non-traumatically". He moved to Europe after losing his job in the aftermath of "*El Corralito*", the 2001 economic depression in Argentina. Once in Europe, he spent a short period of time in Italy before moving to the UK. He was diagnosed with AIDS after getting seriously ill with an opportunistic infection as a result of his damaged immune system.

After starting treatment, his viral load became undetectable, and his CD4 remained high. Two years after his diagnosis, Ramón started therapy because he was feeling lonely and isolated. Having a vague idea that this was related to his health and his HIV status; it was difficult for him to grasp the reasons as he was essentially "a happy man". This "happy man" narrative was recurrent during therapy sessions.

Therapy was in Spanish, and gradually he began introducing sentences in English. His narrative was different when speaking in English, referring, for example, to the shock and disbelief of his diagnosis. He was also surprised he was still alive. Since his teenage years, he had always thought he would die young. I mirrored his use of language and intervened in English or in Spanish following his language choice. Spanish was his mother tongue, but it became evident that he found it easier to express his emotions in English. Problems and difficult emotions were not permitted during his upbringing, and now, speaking in his second language allowed him to explore painful feelings and events while maintaining a certain distance from them.

Bilingual clients may experience an emotional barrier when speaking in their second language. This is because words in a second language hold less emotional weight than the language learnt in childhood. However, "said barrier may, in some cases, help the client to access material so emotionally intense that, otherwise, would provoke excessive anxiety in their native language" (Laguzzi, 2014, p. 37 [My translation]).

After some time of relational and attachment-based therapy, Ramón acknowledged in Spanish the fact that he had been diagnosed on three different occasions: in Argentina, in Italy and in the UK; every time experiencing shock and disbelief. The main apparent difference being the first two diagnoses were HIV and the third was AIDS.

Ramón created his "happy narrative" to disguise the trauma of growing up and discovering his sexual orientation in a heteronormative environment. Under the happy gay man, including partying, casual sexual encounters and drugs in his youth, there was internalised homophobia. His fear of living with HIV was too much of a contradiction with his story to the extreme of denying his two previous diagnoses in order to continue being "happy". When he developed AIDS, his façade started to crumble, and he isolated himself from other gay men and from people living with HIV, from his peers. Therefore, he did not benefit from the resilience and resources that stigmatised groups develop when they are part of their community. At the same time, having AIDS had brought him closer to his belief that he would die young. This belief was probably related to internalised homophobia, and it became almost a self-fulfilling prophecy once he was diagnosed. While Ramón had rational motives to move to different countries, it seemed he was also escaping his ghosts in the shape of consecutive diagnoses. With his consent, I incorporated elements of trauma therapy in our sessions.

He had contacted me after searching for a gay therapist in the Pink Therapy Directory, and his awareness of my sexual orientation was part of the therapeutic process. Clients from gender and sexual diverse groups (GSRD) may experience hypervigilance against prejudice in the therapy room. Because of this, some clients benefit from working with a psychotherapist with the same gender and sexual diversity: "In cases where the therapist's sexual orientation matches the client's and is disclosed, the therapist can sometimes be seen as a role model whether they want that or not" (Cormier-Otaño & Davies, 2012, p. 4).

Ramón related to his HIV status as having the enemy within, and he felt certain contempt towards his equals. Among other interventions, I asked him to draw "his virus" and the importance of perceiving "his HIV" as a friend as it was part of him. He was resistant to it, but eventually, he turned up to his session with a drawing of a smiley face emoji: "this is my HIV". This was just part of his process to make HIV his "friend". Later in the therapy, I told him about a company selling cuddly toys representing different types of microbes, viruses and diseases. I suggested to him to have a look at the toy representing HIV. Eventually he brought it to our session, a cuddly black monster-like figure with big eyes and a red ribbon next to its nose. I asked him to keep bringing it to our sessions, and he would hold it in his lap while talking or when in silence.

The use of a cuddly toy representing HIV comes from the same principles of the Empty Chair Technique used in Gestalt therapy (Kellogg, 2014). When a client experiences an internal conflict, in this case HIV internalised stigma, the personification of HIV in a toy gives the client a visual, physical and tactile representation of the conflicted part within himself. This allows him not only to explore his conflict from a different perspective but also to relate to the part of himself he denies.

By the time therapy ended, Ramón was volunteering for an HIV organisation to continue his healing process. In his case, volunteering was, perhaps, a way of being part of his community while still keeping certain distance from his peers.

The early HIV/AIDS survivors

People diagnosed before or in the early days of ART are the forgotten group. Many saw friends and partners dying from AIDS, and they expected to die young. They may have endured long-term side effects of early treatments, trauma and HIV related stigma at their worst. In 2003, a psychotherapist in an LGBT organisation told me it was possible to know whether somebody had HIV by looking at their face. With this discriminatory remark he was referring to facial fat waste due to lipodystrophy; a long-term side effect of early antiretroviral medication resulting in fat loss or fat gain in different body parts. Fuster-Ruiz de Apodaca et al. (2018) assert, "the type of lipodystrophy, conjointly with certain sociodemographic profiles, is an important factor in an individual's experience of discrimination" (p. 14). Thanks to ART, this demographic has survived and lived after a diagnosis that, at the time, seemed a death sentence. With HIV becoming a chronic condition, they are an "uncomfortable" group (together with some other HIV+ people with comorbidities) because their health, life experiences and trauma don't match policy makers' narrative and criteria.

For many long-term survivors, the COVID-19 pandemic which started in 2020 was reminiscent of the worst times of the HIV pandemic. The lack of knowledge about the new disease and ways of transmission during the pandemic's first months, no effective treatment, the need for social distancing resulting in fear of physical contact, isolation, mistrust in some governments' decisions, guidelines for sexual encounters during the pandemic – all had echoes from the HIV epidemic and its traumatic effects, but also from the resilience and HIV activism developed along the years by different HIV+ communities. Later, in 2022, the emergence of the monkeypox virus became yet again another opportunity for othering gay men and their sexual behaviours as the virus was noticed to spread among that community.

PrEP whore and condom bore

With the HIV epidemic crisis, health practitioners and HIV activists coined and promoted the term safe/safer sex, summarised in the use of condoms for penetrative sex (anal penetration in the case of sex between men). For decades, the use of condoms has been the main preventative tool against HIV and AIDS, with many gay men incorporating and normalising it in their sexual practices.

The term barebacking (originally from the practice of mounting a horse without a saddle) has been referred to as "unsafe" or "unprotected" sex since the 1990s, particularly in relation to anal penetration between men. Actually, barebacking has a deeper connotation than sex without condoms or what is known as condomless sex: it is a conscious decision not to use condoms for anal sex.

Since the 1980s, mainstream gay culture considered condomless penetration reckless or self-harming. In 2018, Alaska and Mario Vaquerizo, two Spanish celebrities, were in a TV programme speaking about an AIDS/HIV charity gala they had attended recently. Referring to people who acquired HIV nowadays, Mario Vaquerizo said:

> You know what's unforgivable? Before, when we didn't have any information, one could be excused, you know what I mean? But, with all the information we have nowadays, it is unforgivable. It is unforgivable because I am not interested in you, because you are a dickhead.
>
> (RETOS VIH 2020, 2018 [My translation])

Alaska added, "It's not justifiable".

Penetration with condoms vs. condomless penetration created a moralistic divide between "good" and "bad" gays. This exacerbated the stigma and preachy approach when a gay man was diagnosed with HIV. He was one of the "bad" gay men who should have known better. As Jaspal (2018) quoted in a series of interviews of HIV negative gay men in the Midlands: "if you end up getting HIV, it's basically down to something you've done. It's stupidity. You can just use a condom, can't you?" (2018, p. 9).

There are myriad reasons why gay men may have or choose to have condomless penetration in their sexual encounters: condom fatigue, difficulty in negotiating sex, low self-esteem, difficulty in maintaining an erection, fear of rejection, assuming sexual partner's HIV status, proof of trust or love, wanting to belong, the heat of the moment, internalised homophobia, feeling liberated, enhanced pleasure, desire for intimacy, or being under the influence of drugs/alcohol, to name a few. Categorising condomless sexual encounters just as reckless demonstrates understanding of neither the complexity of sex and sexual relationships, nor the historic trauma of gay men.

While there are other ways of safer sex, such as mutual masturbation, the message received by the establishment has focused mainly in penetration with condoms, equating, maybe unintentionally, sexual encounters to penetration. This reinforces linear sexual heteronormative formulas and sexual roles whereby many gay men may approach sexual encounters by "what should happen" rather than being led by desire, thus creating sexual dysfunctions. For this, it is relevant to consider some reflections regarding the new *Ars Amandi* [Art of Loving] (Amezúa, 2003). A sexual encounter is the creation between two or more people who desire each other and act on their mutual attraction. In their encounter there are no rules, with key elements being: desire, imagination, curiosity, exploration and craft. Hence, sexual partners create a language that is unique to them and free from formulaic prescriptions.

This reinforcement of heteronormative sexuality was clear in the homophobic initial sentence of a report by NHS England (2016): "PrEP is a measure to prevent HIV transmission, particularly for men who have high risk condomless sex with multiple male partners".

While ART and the use of condoms have been highly effective in preventing HIV, the number of new diagnoses kept increasing among gay men. In the UK, for example, more than half of the new diagnoses were among men who have sex with men (MSM; (Nutland, 2016). Since then, the number of gay men newly diagnosed with HIV in England has plummeted to a twenty-year low (Public Health England, 2020a, 2020b), thanks to starting ART as soon as possible after diagnosis, PrEP, use of condoms, and frequent HIV testing (Public Health England, 2020a).

PrEP consists in taking specific antiretroviral medication as a preventative measure if at high risk of contracting HIV, and it is highly effective when taken as prescribed (there are different ways of taking PrEP safely depending on whether it is for receptive anal penetration – trans and cis men; or receptive vaginal/frontal penetration – trans men). Since 2012, it has slowly been introduced in more than seventy countries, but some of these programmes, particularly in Africa, are not targeting gay men as a high risk group (Avert, 2020).

The concept of safer sex is changing. Hook up and dating gay apps usually have a safer sex field; before U = U and PrEP, the options were basically "Always" (meaning, always condoms), "Never" (meaning bareback), and "It needs discussion" (usually meaning "I'm positive and would like to disclose it when we chat" or "I'm flexible depending on the situation"). Nowadays, many of these apps adapted to gay men's practices whereby, safer sex is not defined by the use of condoms any longer; it is defined by primary and secondary HIV prevention without considering other STIs, with multiple choice options such as: "Condoms", "PrEP", "TasP", "Safe" (without specifying which method) or "Let's discuss".

The use of condoms for penetrative sexual encounters among gay men became normalised as a consequence of the HIV epidemic. Now that there are other preventative measures, it would make sense that some men choose condomless sex. This is problematic for some people because condoms are the most effective protection against other STIs. Still, there are numerous instances of transmission of other STIs during sexual encounters involving condoms. This is because of the possibility of contracting specific STIs during other sexual practices such as rimming, fingering, water sports, fisting or oral sex. Individuals on PrEP get regular sexual health check-ups to receive their prescriptions.

Bareback sexual encounters are becoming mainstream (Levine, 2021). As a colleague sexual health nurse told me discussing gay men on PrEP: "once they have tried without condoms, there is no way back". Many gay men on PrEP decrease their use of condoms but still may choose to use them in situations where they feel particularly vulnerable to other STIs, such as group sex, or when their sexual partner prefers using condoms. The old "good" and "bad" gay men divide has evolved into what Knoll and Geiger (2019) call *PrEP-Schlampen* and *Kondom-Langweiler* (Prep Whore and Condom Bore). Some individuals on PrEP or TasP as the only preventative measure consider themselves up-to-date with new means of safer sex while perceiving condom users as yesteryear. Meanwhile, some people who choose condom use may consider PrEP users and people who use TasP as the only secondary prevention to be reckless or sluts. Safer sex is no longer one size fits all, and together with new possibilities, old and new stigmas and dynamics develop within gay communities. To avoid rejection, some men might experience peer pressure to bareback because a potential sexual partner is on PrEP. A client recalled how, at times, he used to engage in condomless sex in the heat of the moment. He would then feel guilty and experience those instances as a way of self-harming. Now, as a PrEP user, he chooses when to bareback and when to use condoms. On reflection, he believes his feeling of self-harming was out of guilt, and on PrEP he feels empowered.

ART and PrEP are also changing serosorting. Serosorting consists in choosing sexual or romantic partners only with the same HIV status. Now, like the safer sex concept, this is becoming more complex with gay men choosing sexual partners depending on both HIV status and/or means of protection: negative, positive, undetectable, condoms, TasP or PrEP.

Before ART, some sexual practices remained hidden or underground. Now different approaches towards sexual exploration, queer identities and masculinities are becoming more visible. Examples of this would be the hyper-masculinisation of "getting fucked among gay pigs" (Florêncio, 2020) whereby "you take it like a man", or the eroticisation and exchange of all kinds of body fluids and secretions in different practices, particularly in group sex scenarios.

HIV becoming a chronic condition has meant that many health professionals and psychotherapists have not kept informed about the changes and developments around HIV, including treatments, prevention and attitudes. Some therapists, including those who promote themselves as LGBTQ positive, may approach it as a non-issue when it is and as an issue when it isn't; thus failing clients. Lack of knowledge might act as a barrier in the alliance with our clients.

On one occasion, Jordi recounted during a session how a previous psychotherapist was set aback when he told him he was having condomless penetration with his partner, who was HIV positive with an undetectable viral load. Jordi felt defensive and had to explain that, according to sexual health professionals, it was safe for them to have condomless sex. "There is always a possibility of catching it if you have unsafe sex" was his therapist's reply.

It is sometimes reasonable for a client explaining something their therapist doesn't know. This wasn't one of those moments. This client felt betrayed by his therapist's judgement and inaccurate knowledge, particularly because he contacted him as an LGBTQ inclusive psychotherapist. The alliance broke, and Jordi ended his therapy a few sessions later. This therapist, with his outdated knowledge and prejudice, shamed his client, creating an issue where there was none, thus reinforcing the stigma associated with HIV and gay sexuality. His lack of knowledge could have been solved with honesty rather than judgement: "I'm not up-to-date with safer sex practices in relation to serodiscordant couples", "how is it for you barebacking with your partner?" or just remaining in silence and continuing listening could have been valid interventions.

Serodiscordant relationships are those couples in which each partner has a different HIV status. If the positive partner has an undetectable viral load thanks to ART, they can choose condomless sex. If the HIV+ partner has a detectable viral load, they have the option of either using condoms or for the HIV negative partner to take PrEP.

Case 2

Two middle aged gay cis men, Will and John, had been in a monogamous relationship for seven years. They came to therapy because of Will's erectile dysfunction. His presentation started "a few years ago" and only in their sexual encounters. He had no erection problems when masturbating. As a consequence, they were struggling with intimacy with each other as, according to them, their sexual encounters were now loaded by expectations and anxiety.

After a few sessions, they explained that when they started their relationship both were living with HIV, but later on John learnt he had been misdiagnosed. He was diagnosed with HIV ten years earlier during a work trip abroad. After being arrested due to an altercation while high on illegal drugs and taken to hospital for examination, he was brought in front of a judge. During the hearing, together with the altercation details, they reported his HIV positive status. This was how he learnt he was HIV+.

On his return to the UK, John, deeply distressed, continued with his life without acting on his new diagnosis. Three years later, John and Will met and started their relationship. Because both had HIV, they "didn't need to worry about that". Two years later, John finally went to his hospital for his HIV to be monitored and start treatment if appropriate. To start the process, they tested his blood, and he was shocked by the results: he did not have HIV. To this day he doesn't know why he was misinformed he was HIV+ at the hearing, but he believes it was prejudice: "a foreign gay guy high on drugs and involved in a fight sounds even worse if he has HIV".

John and Will never discussed in depth what this meant for their relationship. When they started dating, their HIV status was relevant because Will was serosorting. He had previously experienced rejection due to his HIV status, so he wanted a partner also with HIV. John had being single since "becoming positive", and dating another man with HIV had helped him greatly coming to terms with his (unknowingly yet) misdiagnosis. During therapy, Will acknowledged that if he had known John was HIV negative, he wouldn't have started dating him. Their unexpected different status had shaken their relationship dynamics, and this had not been addressed.

Because of Will's experiences of HIV related stigma, after discovering John was HIV negative, he gradually started feeling dirty and ashamed in his sexual encounters with his partner, and this process was unconscious. When John realised his misdiagnosis, he started taking PrEP. This is not medically needed if your partner's viral load is undetectable, but some people in serodiscordant relationships decide to take it because they find it empowering: "He does his bit with TasP and I do my bit with PrEP", John explained. Still, his motives to take PrEP had not been discussed at the time, thus reinforcing Will's shame and the unconscious belief that John needed to protect himself from his partner. Will mitigated his shame by developing erectile dysfunction in their sexual encounters. Meanwhile, John received Will's lack of erection as rejection and felt undesired. He was confusing desire with arousal.

Once these issues became conscious and they started untangling them, I started introducing non-demand and other type of exploratory intimacy encounters. They agreed to an artist/sitter life drawing experience, alternating these roles in two different encounters. The "sitter" poses in the nude, while the "artist" covers the paper where he is drawing, thus he is unable to see his own sketching. This experience mirrors some elements in sexual encounters; exploring intimacy and connection without physical contact. This exercise is designed so that, while being outside their comfort zone, it is safe by them setting up the exercise boundaries. The setup parameters allow them to gain insight to what they usually bring to their sexual encounters. They both might feel vulnerable, with the "sitter" being the subject of attention without reciprocating, and the "artist" unable to "succeed" in producing a "good drawing". The aim is the experience per se, with the end drawing being irrelevant, challenging linear conceptions of sexual encounters and exploring being present, anxiety performance, expectations, and sexual roles. During one of these drawing exercises, Will was surprised by his own arousal; later, in the therapy room, they discussed his arousal and their dynamics during the experience. The use of creativity in these exercises was useful to introduce in therapy concepts from the new *Ars Amandi* mentioned earlier. When therapy ended, their sexual intimacy was freer from HIV related stigma, and they were more erotically self-aware.

Note on case 2

It could be argued I should enquire about gay clients' HIV status in the initial form they complete when starting therapy or, at the very least, during the initial consultation. At the end of the day, it is estimated that one in eight gay men in London live with HIV. Not requesting this information is a therapeutic decision. On one hand, clients start therapy with their own anxieties and asking possible unrelated information before the start of the therapeutic process is invasive and related more to therapists' anxiety than to the benefit of clients. On the other hand,

I choose not to collude with the association between being gay and HIV. While in this case HIV was relevant, on many other presentations, clients' HIV status is not. The initial form I have for clients is specifically about health and safety and the suitability of starting therapy.

Conclusions

The limitations of this chapter are laid out in its title: "The impact of antiretroviral therapies and PrEP on gay men". Therefore, this text would apply to gay men living in places where both TasP and PrEP are widely available to them, which is, for the most part, wealthy countries or urban areas where gay men can access free or affordable sexual health services without homophobic and HIV related stigma discrimination.

HIV transmission among gay men is being reduced dramatically in those countries in which ART and PrEP have been effectively implemented. Gay men's fear of HIV is decreasing, and the association between desire, gay sexuality and death has started to diminish. With the new preventative measures, the use of condoms and the concept of safer sex are changing. Many gay men are feeling able to explore their sexuality in ways they thought impossible during the hardest

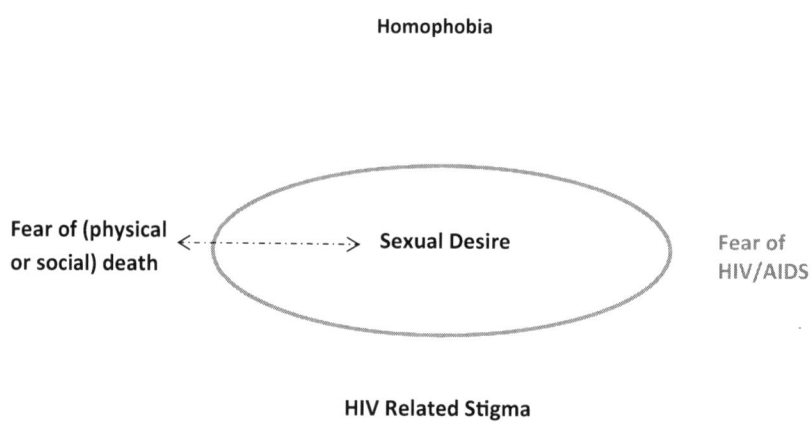

Homophobia

Fear of (physical or social) death <----------> **Sexual Desire**   Fear of HIV/AIDS

HIV Related Stigma

Trauma in Gay Men

after ART and PrEP implementation

Figure 11.2 Trauma in gay men after ART and PrEP implementation.

years of the epidemic: "it's like being in 1979 again", a client on PrEP told me recently. Having said that, both homophobia and HIV related stigma continue to be prominent in society and within gay communities. This makes the total break up between gay sexual desire and death impossible (Figure 11.2). ART has been a life changer for people with HIV, but to this day, there is no cure for HIV.

Further reading

Ashford, C., Morris, M., & Powell, A. (2020). Bareback sex in the age of preventative medication: Rethinking the 'harms' of HIV transmission. *The Journal of Criminal Law*, *84*(6), 596–614.

Grace, D., Jollimore, J., MacPherson, P., Strang, M. J. P., & Tan, D. H. S. (2018). The pre-exposure prophylaxis-stigma paradox: Learning from Canada's first wave of PrEP users. *AIDS Patient Care STDS*, *32*(1), 24–30.

HIV Psychosocial Network. (2018). *Ten Years After: An 'Austerity Audit' of Services and Living Conditions for People Living with HIV in the UK, a Decade after the Financial Crisis*. Retrieved December 15, 2022, from www.hivpsychosocialnetwork.wordpress.com/the-10-years-after-austerity-audit-report/

Méndez, M. (2018). El VIH y la proximidad corporal. Sexo, amor y silencio entre varones gay. [HIV and Body Proximity. Sex, love and silence among gay men]. *Sexualidad, Salud y Sociedad (Rio de Janeiro)*, 159–177. http://doi.org/10.1590/1984-6487.sess.2018.28.09.a

Squire, C. (2010). Being naturalised, being left behind: The HIV citizen in the era of treatment possibility. *Critical Public Health*, *20*(4), 401–427.

Wilberg, M. (2021). *HIV and condom use down, STIs up: The impact of U=U and PrEP at a clinic in Seattle*. Washington. Retrieved September 13, 2021, from www.aidsmap.com/news/aug-2021/hiv-and-condom-use-down-stis-impact-uu-and-prep-clinic-seattle-washington

Williamson, I., Papaloukas, P., Jaspal, R., & Lond, B. (2019). 'There's this glorious pill': Gay and bisexual men in the English midlands navigate risk responsibility and pre-exposure prophylaxis. *Critical Public Health*, *29*(5), 560–571.

Young, I., Davis, M., Flowers, P., & McDaid, L. (2019). Navigating HIV citizenship: Identities, risks and biological citizenship in the treatment as prevention era. *Health, Risk & Society*, *21*(1–2), 1–16.

Zimmermann, H. M. L., Jongen, V. W., Boyd, A., Hoornenborg, E., Prins, M., de Vries, H. J. C., Schim van der Loeff, M. F., & Davidovich, U. (2020). Decision-making regarding condom use among daily and event-driven users of preexposure prophylaxis in the Netherlands. *AIDS*, *34*(15), 2295–2304.

References

Alessi, E. J., Martin, J. I., Gyamerah, A., & Meyer, I. H. (2013). Prejudice events and traumatic stress among heterosexuals and lesbians, gay men and bisexuals. *Journal of Aggression, Maltreatment & Trauma*, *22*(5). http://doi.org/10.1080/10926771.2013.785455

American Psychiatric Association. (2013). *Diagnostic and Statistical Manual of Mental Disorders: DSM-5* (5th ed.). Washington, DC: American Psychiatric Publishing.

Amezúa, E. (2003). El sexo: historia de una idea [Sex: History of an Idea] Revista española de sexología. *Instituto de Sexología*, 115–116.

Avert. (2020). *Pre-Exposure Prophylaxis (Prep) for HIV Prevention*. Retrieved August 25, 2021, from www.avert.org/professionals/hiv-programming/prevention/pre-exposure-prophylaxis

Bolton, R. (1992). AIDS and promiscuity: Muddles in the models of HIV prevention. *Medical Anthropology, 14*(2–4), 145–223.

Carrascosa, S., & Sáez, J. (2011). *Por el culo. Políticas anales* [Up the Arse. Anal Politics]. Egales. Madrid-Barcelona.

Caswell, T. A., & Sackett-Fox, K. (2018). Gender-atypical personality or sexual behavior: What is disgusting about male homosexuality? *The Journal of Social Psychology, 158*(5), 591–602.

Catalan, J., Hedge, B., & Ridge, D. (2020). *HIV in the UK: Voices from the Epidemic*. Abingdon, NY: Routledge.

Collins English Dictionary. (2018). Retrieved July 15, 2021, from www.collinsdictionary.com/dictionary/masculine

Cormier-Otaño, O., & Davies, D. (2012). *Gender and Sexual Diversity Therapy (GSDT)*. Retrieved September 1, 2021, from www.pinktherapy.com/Portals/0/Downloadables/Translations/GB_GSDT.pdf

Crewe, T. (2018). Here was a plague. *The London Review of Books, 40*(18). Retrieved June 20, 2021, from www.lrb.co.uk/the-paper/v40/n18/tom-crewe/here-was-a-plague

Eisinger, R. W., Dieffenbach, C. W., & Fauci, A. S. (2019). HIV viral load and transmissibility of HIV infection: Undetectable equals untransmittable. *JAMA, 321*(5), 451–452.

Florêncio, J. (2020). *Bareback Porn, Porous Masculinities, Queer Futures. The Ethics of Becoming-Pig*. Abingdon, NY: Routledge.

Fuster-Ruiz de Apodaca, M. J., Molero, F., Sansinenea, E., Holgado, F.-P., Magallares, A., & Agirrezabal, A. (2018). Discriminación percibida, autoexclusión y bienestar entre las personas con VIH en función de los síntomas de la lipodistrofia [Perceived discrimination, self-exclusion and well-being among people with HIV as a function of lipodystrophy symptoms]. *Anales de Psicología, 34*(1), 7–15.

Jaspal, R. (2018). HIV and gay men in the era of antiretroviral therapy. *Psychology of Sexualities Review, 9*(2), 2–15. ISSN 2047-1467.

Kellogg, S. (2014). *Transformational Chairwork. Using Psychotherapeutic Dialogues in Clinical Practice*. Lanham, MD: Roman & Littlefield.

Knoll, C., & Geiger, J. (2019). Wo ist das Kondom geblieben? [Where have all the condoms gone?]. *MMW – Fortschritte der Medizin, 161*, 25–26.

Laguzzi, A. L. (2014). Bilingüismo y Psicoterapia [Bilinguism and psychotherapy]. *Psicodebate, 14*(1), 33–44.

Levine, N. (2021). *'Raw Is Law' – How Anal Sex Without Condoms Is Going Mainstream*. Retrieved September 13, 2021, from www.vice.com/en/article/xgz5gj/how-bareback-sex-went-mainstream

Meyer, I. H. (2003). Prejudice, social stress, and mental health in lesbian, gay, and bisexual populations: Conceptual issues and research evidence. *Psychological bulletin, 129*(5), 674–697.

Morrison, T. G., Kiss, M. J., Bishop, C. J., & Morrison, M. A. (2019). We're disgusted with queers, not fearful of them: The interrelationships among disgust, gay men's sexual behavior, and homonegativity. *Journal of Homosexuality, 66*(7), 1014–1033.

NHS England. (2016). *August Update on the Commissioning and Provision of Pre Exposure Prophylaxis (PREP) for HIV Prevention*. Retrieved September 7, 2021, from www.england.nhs.uk/2016/08/august-update-on-the-commissioning-and-provision-of-pre-exposure-prophylaxis-prep-for-hiv-prevention/

Nutland, W. (2016). *The Acceptability of Pre-Exposure HIV Prophylaxis in Men Who Have Sex with Men in London*. DrPH thesis, London School of Hygiene & Tropical Medicine.

Pachankis, J. E., Clark, K. A., Burton, C. L., Hughto, J., Bränström, R., & Keene, D. E. (2020). Sex, status, competition, and exclusion: Intraminority stress from within the gay community and gay and bisexual men's mental health. *Journal of Personality and Social Psychology, 119*(3), 713–740.

Public Health England. (2020a). *New HIV Diagnoses in Gay and Bisexual Men at Their Lowest in 20 Years* [Press release]. Retrieved July 13, 2021 from www.gov.uk/government/news/new-hiv-diagnoses-in-gay-and-bisexual-men-at-their-lowest-in-20-years

Public Health England. (2020b). Trends in HIV testing, new diagnoses and people receiving HIV-related care in the UK: Data to end December 2019. *Health Protection Report, 14*(20).

RETOS VIH 2020. (2018, November 21). *#STOPSTIGMA*. Retrieved June 14, 2021, from www.youtube.com/watch?v=x9gdj_h5TqE

Rothschild, B. (2000). *The Body Remembers. The Psychophysiology of Trauma and Trauma Treatment*. New York: W.W. Norton & Company.

Chapter 12

GSRD-affirmative supervision of psychotherapy

Dr Daniel Bąk

Introduction

"Supervision, the foundation of clinical development, is one of the most important and influential processes in the personal and professional growth of a clinician" (Resnick & Estrup, 2000, p. 121). Indeed, aimed at supporting the client–supervisee relationship, supervision extraordinarily contributes to the advancement of the supervisee's personal and professional clinical competencies (Gilbert & Evans, 2000). It is due to the numerous purposes embraced by the supervisory process (Resnick & Estrup, 2000; modified by the author):

1   Supporting the supervisee in better understanding of the client at both the content and processual levels.
2   Supporting the supervisee's awareness of their reactions to the client – the actual ones in the here-and-now, and those being the enduring relational themes of the supervisee (Jacobs, 2017a).
3   Supporting the clinical and theoretical understanding of the client–supervisee contact dynamics.
4   Looking at the supervisee's interventions and understanding their clinical and relational consequences.
5   Comparing and learning of different psychotherapy theories.
6   Broadening the supervisee's repertoire of ways of working (other psychotherapy models).
7   Both supporting and challenging the supervisee.

From summarising different goals of supervision, at least three possible roles of the supervisor emerge (Chidiac et al., 2017): an ethical and legal gatekeeper to ensure professional standards (it actually permeates all of the aforementioned: 1–7, but especially: 2–4), a trainer (especially: 4–6) and mentor (especially: 7).

Supervision is a complex amalgamate of tasks and goals in which the clinical realm is seen through many different lenses (Resnick & Estrup, 2000; modified by the author):

DOI: 10.4324/9781003260561-13

1   Personality functioning of the client, supervisee, and supervisor.
2   The client–supervisee and the supervisee–supervisor relationships.
3   The wider context of all supervision parties (the client, supervisee, supervisor) and of their relationships, be it culture, politics, or important intersections of gender, sexuality, age, spirituality, etc.
4   Psychotherapeutic theories in use, especially theories of development.
5   Diagnosis (medical, characterological, phenomenological).
6   Treatment.
7   Professional, especially ethical and legal gate-keeping.
8   Administration and business.

This complexity needs a theoretical model which takes into account the multi-dimensional nature of the supervisory process and supports the supervisee and supervisor in staying attuned to the intricacies of supervision. In this chapter, the Relational Matrix Model (RMM) – authored by Marie-Anne Chidiac et al. (2017) – is presented. The model is an original conceptualisation of supervision, drawing from and developing the work of Peter Hawkins and Robin Shohet (1989, 2006) as well as Michael Caroll and Maria C. Gilbert (2011). The model's stance is immensely relational, and special significance is ascribed to the contextual dimensions of supervision.

Specificities of this chapter

The Relational Matrix Model was created by Gestalt theorists and practitioners working as supervisors in many different contexts, including coaching, psychotherapy, counselling, consulting, management, and training (Chidiac et al., 2017). The model rests on modern, relational Gestalt theory being a contemporary elaboration of core Gestalt concepts such as field theory, self-process, and phenomenology. However, being *of* Gestalt theory, the RMM can be considered a meta-model of supervision. The focus of the RMM is not on Gestalt principles themselves, but rather on the specific modes of clinical thinking and quality of the supervisory relationship that need to be fostered in supervision. As a consequence, theoretical orientations of the supervisor and supervisee should not be limiting factors in making use of the RMM.

The Relational Matrix Model is a general model of supervision. Nonetheless, in this chapter, its application in a GSRD-affirmative manner will be discussed. After introducing the RMM's structure, particular attention will be given to GSRD issues in supervision. Detailed elaboration of the RMM, with less specialised examples of use, can be found elsewhere (Chidiac et al., 2017).

The good of the client is the main subject and goal of the supervisory process (Gilbert & Evans, 2000). In the author's experience, two key GSRD-specific factors hugely influence psychotherapy with GSRD clients: (1) their level of GSRD identity self-acceptance and (2) the extent of external oppression suffered by a GSRD individual due to their gender, sexual, and/or relationship identity. These two components – supporting a GSRD client's self-acceptance and taking external oppression into account – will be the focal points when translating the RMM's structure and principles into a GSRD-affirmative and GSRD-knowledgeable tool. It will be examined what supervisee's/supervisor's attitudes, thinking, and interventions support or impede the client's self-process in the discriminatory environment. Importantly, it is not only the client's non-heteronormative identity that can "make" supervision GSRD-affirmative. The impact of the supervisee's or supervisor's GSRD identity on support opportunities with GSRD clients will also be discussed.

Relationality is a basic and profound organising meta-principle in the RMM, increasingly well-grounded in neuroscience (Clark-Polner & Clark, 2014; Mizen & Hook, 2020) and contemporary psychotherapeutic theories (Hayes, 2004; Jacobs & Hycner, 2009; Safran & Kraus, 2015; Wachtel, 2010). Before introducing the RMM itself, basic tenets of the relational approach in psychotherapy and supervision will be reminded, with a special focus on their value when working in the GSRD context.

Relational approach in psychotherapy and supervision

Lynne Jacobs summarises four foundational assumptions on relationality.

> First and foremost, our relationality is irreducible. Our relatedness in our environment and with each other does not begin with us as separate selves, with relatedness being an "add-on". Our very existence is utterly, thoroughly context-dependent, and our worlds of experience are emergent from our contexts. We have no experience that is prior to relatedness. (. . .) Every experience we have, including that right now, between us, is co-shaped, or co-emergent from what I bring and what you bring, along with our setting, our task, and other aspects that go into comprising our situation. Your emergent subjectivity and mine are utterly interdependent.
>
> (2009, p. 44)

Secondly, she continues with the realisation about all of us being more alike than not. We are born into a shared context of being human, which makes us similar in terms of using a meaningful language, our carnality, or neurobiological readiness to resonate and communicate with each other. Thirdly, she notices that what we have in common makes the connection between us possible. However, these are our individual characteristics which make contacting interesting, give the relationship "a breath of fresh air", and create an opportunity for all parties to learn something new. Fourthly, she indicates that our sense of self, encompassing such dimensions as a sense of agency, emotional capacities, individuation, or capacity for intimacy, rely on our past (developmental) and current emotional contexts.

The aforementioned assumptions on relationality result in important clinical consequences and suggestions (Jacobs, 2009). They can be operationalised as three main relational topics: co-emergence, confirmation and attunement, and relational moral stance.

Co-emergence describes a situation in which whatever happens in the consulting room results from what happens "between" the client and therapist or the supervisee and supervisor. Nothing that happens arises solely, for example, from "within" the supervisee and "within" the supervisor. From such a theoretical position, concepts like (counter)transference or projection need to be renounced as relics of an individualistic and non-relational approach. The relational supervisor, who understands co-emergent phenomena, would rather think: "Something is happening between us, what brings these specific experiences to me and my supervisee. I am not sure what it is". The only way to try to untangle this contact complexity would be to engage in a dialogue with the supervisee; a dialogue characterised by "the horizontalism of phenomenological exploration" (Jacobs, 2009, p. 49). It means that the supervisee would be considered the source of true self, as someone who has meaningful information about themselves and the supervisory situation, on par with the supervisor. Noteworthily, this dialogue would be an interaction of two subjectivities (intersubjectivity; Stolorow et al., 1994) because the supervisee's and supervisor's experiences – particularly feelings, a sense of knowledge, and embodied quality of their "between" in the supervisory situation – are co-emergent phenomena of their separate experiential fields.

The supervisee and supervisor meet on the common ground, which can be diverse in the case of different supervisory relationships, and make the meeting possible: a mutual interest in learning/teaching encounter, theoretical orientation, age, gender, or sexual identity (e.g. the supervisee and supervisor being both gestaltists, middle-aged, cis-males, and gay). Simultaneously, their meeting can be enriching for both parts since they bring their unique phenomenological fields into the relationship – above all, their ways of exploring, experiencing, and embodying a therapeutic/supervisory situation, shaped (without one's awareness) by the context of their personal histories, language, culture, politics, etc. One ought to remember that our phenomenological fields, however unique, are actually shared fields. It is because some common contextual aspects, such as language or culture, may result in "islands" of shared experience. This fields' overlapping is most obvious with situations of you-being-in-my-world and me-being-in-your-world, which are basic constituents of inclusion (Jacobs, 2004) – this key quality of the supervisee's and supervisor's work in the relational model (Gilbert & Evans, 2000).

As it was mentioned previously, our sense of self depends on the past and current emotional contexts. It implies that "not only is the quality of our contacting a co-emergent process, but the developmental trajectory of our patients relies on the quality of the relational supports for development that inhere in the therapeutic relationship" (Jacobs, 2009, p. 47). It can be reasonably hypothesised that this statement is also true for the supervisee and the supervisory relationship. Jacobs (2009) points out emotional availability, understood as emotional attunement and emotional responsiveness, being one of the crucial relational supports. Attunement seems to operate in two ways. On the one hand, its function is regulatory. People, by attuning to each other, are able to co-regulate their emotional states in a dialogue since attunement enhances a sense of affect validity, expression, and integration. But attunement is also an attempt to recognise the wholeness of the client or supervisee. By trying to stay attuned to the client or supervisee, we hope to come closer and embrace their emotional life, shaped by the context of the past and the present. In this recognition of a unique, yet intelligible person, there is an act of existential confirmation: "When I meet them (clients; the author's note), they are confirmed as both a contributing and understandable other in the stream of human relatedness. This is a restoration of dignity, and the restoration of dignity is transformative confirmation" (Jacobs, 2009, p. 52).

The last issue is a moral stance beyond the relational approach. Jacobs (2009, p. 47) refers to "visionary sensibility" amplified by focusing on innate relatedness of the world. Indeed, as co-shapers of our own and others' life contexts, we should ask ourselves some important questions. What kind of social world do I want to help to co-create? How do I contribute to the othering process of those who feel marginalised? What kind of togetherness do I want to co-create? With these questions, shared responsibility for others and for the world emerges. Furthermore, these questions bring easily to mind the socio-cultural oppression of GSRD people.

The relational approach as the key methodology with GSRD issues

We live in the global, constantly changing world of interconnectedness between people, institutions, and ideas. The relational approach offers us a psychotherapeutic methodology to untangle this complexity. Three key, mentioned before, relational topics – co-emergence, attunement, and relational moral stance (Jacobs, 2009) – can be exceptionally helpful in better understanding of GSRD experiences. They can also provide practical guidance when working with GSRD clients and supervisees.

GSRD experiences are co-emergent phenomena. What happens to a GSRD person is not only a function of what is "within" the person but also of their life context. For instance, a client or supervisee being a cis-woman, lesbian, and Asian may encounter different reactions from their cis-man, heterosexual, and white therapist/supervisor, depending on the therapist's/supervisor's attitudes towards gender, sexual identity, and race. It is clear that relational focus may sensitise mental health professionals to different forms of social oppression present in the field, be it homo-, bi-, transphobia, racism, ageism, or classism. Not to be missed, the oppressor in the client's/supervisee's field can be the therapist/supervisor themselves. Relational stance invites also reflection amongst socially privileged professionals on how their privilege(s) co-shape their work with clients. Appreciating intersectionality harmonises easily with the relational approach.

As mentioned before, according to Jacobs (2009), attunement in a relationship is an act of recognition – an attempt to recognise one's wholeness as a human being. Peter Baumann (2007) says that receiving recognition is a very basic human need, and giving it – a sign of respect in front of the other. Refusal or withdrawal of this very elementary form of respect is in itself a violation of one's dignity. Drawing from Baumann's work, Jacobs (2017b) asserts that what brings clients to the consulting room most often are attacks on their dignity. It must be the case with GSRD individuals. Instead of being recognised as valid human beings with their emotions, unique life narratives, needs, and vulnerabilities, GSRD clients, supervisees, and supervisors suffer from being oppressed. Far too often, they experience physical violence, humiliation, and shaming and are dehumanised because of their nonheteronormative identity. Undoubtedly, this hurtful situation should be a call for action, also among supervisees and supervisors, those who are GSRD or not.

The relational approach makes us co-responsible for relationships we co-create and for the world we co-shape. For example, for those being supervisors, inescapable questions arise: What kind of the supervisory environment I want to create for my supervisees: GSRD-aware and -affirmative or GSRD-phobic and -oppressive? What kind of a dialogue around gender and sexuality do I want to model for my supervisees (and their clients)? Solving these dilemmas requires directing the supervisor's awareness towards the personal (e.g. "Through my life history, I am apprehensive of differences between me and others".) as well as to the socio-political domain of the wider field (e.g. "Being privileged for my cis-genderness, am I aware enough of trans-oppression in my country? What could trans-oppression actually mean?"). The supervisor, who teaches the supervisee how to look at the supervisory and therapeutic relationships through both the personal and socio-political lenses, becomes a psychosocial activist. Jack Aylward (2018) created this term to describe the therapist's attitude of acknowledgment of the personal in the client, on par with the socio-political in the client's life context, to understand the client's psychological difficulties fully. This type of therapist's engagement may result in interventions designed to change the client's environment with the client's hands. This way, what has been disturbed through the environmental influences can be gradually healed. In the author's opinion, the term "a psychosocial activist" can reasonably be used to describe the supervisee, and the supervisor as well. How social and political issues inhere in the psychotherapy field can be found elsewhere (Bąk, 2021).

All the aforementioned complexity of supervision itself, combined with demands originating from GSRD specificity, needs a model containing such multidimensionality. It is proposed that the RMM gives an efficient theoretical frame for this.

The relational matrix model of supervision

Key understandings of the relational approach were summarised by Sally Denham-Vaughan and Marie-Anne Chidiac as the SOS model, where "SOS" stands for "Self, Other, and Situation" (2013). The model highlights interrelatedness of the following elements:

1 Self – an individual, organisation, a group, or community.
2 Other – "the other" in the relationship at any given moment. It is important to notice that it can also be "the other within the self". For instance, the internalised therapist or supervisor.
3 Situation – the overall context from which the issues emerge.

It is assumed that

> when the three processes of Self, Other and Situation are all operating in ways that respond to the demand qualities of the context, then we are most "present"; able to access our fullest potential in accordance with our most deeply held values.
>
> (Chidiac et al., 2017, p. 23)

	CLIENT	SUPERVISEE (Therapist/ Coach, etc.)	SUPERVISOR
SELF	**1** • Focus on the client, their narrative, presenting issue and self support.	**4** • Focus on the supervisee, their experiences and self support.	**7** • Focus on the supervisor, their experiences and self support.
OTHER (Relational field)	**2** • Focus on client relationships (key relational supports in varying contexts). • Focus on relationship of coaching client with organisation.	**5** • Focus on the relationship between the supervisee and client. • Focus on strategies and interventions used by supervisee in their work.	**8** • Focus on supervisory relationship including parallel processes, co-transference, etc.
SITUATION (Wider relational context)	**3** • Wider client field context and culture. • Wider organisational context and culture (e.g. in coaching case).	**6** • Focus on supervisee and client field, including contracting, professional & ethical codes, cultural and situational context. • Focus on relationship of supervisee with client's organisation (if relevant).	**9** • Focus on supervisory field generally, including contracting, professional & ethical codes, cultural and situational context. • Focus on supervisor links with client context e.g. 3rd party contract (if applicable).

Figure 12.1 Relational matrix model of supervision.

Source: Courtesy of Marie-Anne Chidiac, Sally Denham-Vaughan, and Lynda Osborne

From combining the SOS model's components with dimensions of the client, supervisee, and supervisor, the Relational Matrix Model arises (Figure 12.1). It consists of nine interrelated areas of inquiry – "cells". Every cell refers to a different aspect of the supervisory process (Chidiac et al., 2017; modified by the author):

- Cell 1: The Client in Focus (Client x Self); this cell focuses on the client, their presentation (the way they speak, breathe, sit, their facial expression), the narratives they bring, the issues they would like to explore and resolve. The cell invites the supervisee to get interested in the client's process. Importantly, some supervisees are stuck in this cell, reporting on the client in a very detailed manner, overlooking the wider perspective typical of the following cells.
- Cell 2: The Client's Key Relational Supports (Client x Other); in this cell, attention is directed towards key, past and present, client's relationships. It is explored which of them were/are/could potentially be the client's relational support sources. Furthermore, the client's endured relational themes are investigated here.
- Cell 3: The Wider Client's Field (Client x Situation); this cell focuses on the client's wider context, be it the culture they live in, religion or spirituality they adhere to, or political milieu in their country. The task here is to stay curious about the impact of the wider field on the client's presenting issues. Significantly, the supervisee's and/or supervisor's prejudices and stereotypes may thwart such a curious exploration.
- Cell 4: The Supervisee in Focus (Supervisee x Self); in this cell, attention shifts towards the supervisee: their level of professional development, learning style, and theoretical orientation. However, the supervisee's more personal attitudes are explored as well: specific strengths, vulnerabilities, and self-supports. It allows acknowledging the supervisee's unique personhood, which can influence contact processes with both the client and supervisor.
- Cell 5: The Supervisee and Client Relationship (Supervisee x Other); two different aspects of the client–supervisee relationship are in focus in this cell. Firstly, strategies and interventions being employed by the supervisee when working with the client. Secondly, what is "between" the supervisee and client becomes of interest here. Co-emergent phenomena in their relationship are explored, as well as endured relational themes on both sides.
- Cell 6: The Supervisee and Client Field (Supervisee x Situation); this cell directs attention towards the contextual factors of the wider field that co-shape the client–supervisee relationship. Details of the contract between the supervisee and client would be explored here. Moreover, the legal and ethical context of therapeutic work is carefully considered in this cell, for instance: ethical codes and guidelines, specific resolutions, position statements, and operational policies.

- Cell 7: The Supervisor in Focus (Supervisor x Self); in this cell, the supervisor stays in the spotlight. Their professional as well as personal attitudes – which can support or interfere with the supervisory relationship – are taken into consideration.
- Cell 8: The Supervisory Relationship (Supervisor x Other); in this cell, building and maintaining the effective supervisory alliance is attentively approached. Importantly, co-emergent phenomena of parallel processes are looked at here. Through mutual resolving of the field between the supervisee and supervisor, the awareness of the parallel processes may arise, giving key insights into what is happening between the supervisee and client.
- Cell 9: The Supervisory Field (Supervisor x Situation); in this cell, a professional context of supervision is in focus. For example: mindful contracting (also three- or even four-handed contracts with their complexities), dual relationships, and ethical codes declared by the supervisor are relevant here.

The RMM's structure is considered to consist of two distinct parts. The first one covers cells 1, 2, 3, 6, and 9. This L-shaped area indicates aspects of the supervisory process being the ground from which supervisory figures emerge. It is suggested that what is figural in supervision is covered by cells 4, 5, 7, and 8. The RMM's authors advise that this lens of figure/ground is useful for the supervisor to observe where they spend most of the time in supervision. Frequently, the supervisor and supervisee occupy primarily "the figure cells" with the feeling of "real work" being done, while only through acknowledgment of "the ground cells" can the figural in supervision be understood fully (Chidiac et al., 2017).

The next section discusses the application of the RMM to GSRD-affirmative supervision.

GSRD-affirmative supervision and the RMM

In this section, the RMM is translated into a GSRD-affirmative supervisory tool. Firstly, the RMM's cells are discussed afresh, but this time specifically through the GSRD lens:

- Cell 1: Client x Self; in this cell, the client's process around a GSRD identity, be it – for example – bisexual, genderqueer, or polyamorous, is in focus. The client's GSRD identity is informative of specific prejudice and stereotypes operating in the client's life due to their non-heteronormativity; moreover, the personal and institutional consequences of oppression should also become clearer. Is it easy for the client to find a sexual and/or romantic partner? Is the client allowed to become a parent or spouse? Noteworthily, although oppression tools may be the same, like microaggressions, physical violence, or institutionalised hatred, such cognitive and emotional attitudes as homo-, bi-, and transphobia are separate phenomena. It is because they emerge from overlapping, though nonidentical sets of stereotypes.

Broadening the supervisee's and supervisor's awareness in this cell enables them also to see the client as an embodied GSRD person. GSRD-targeted oppression is being inscribed into GSRD bodies. In my experience, it is likely to manifest, for example, as the client's inability to talk about their gender and/or sexuality (the larynx becomes speechless), sexual issues (e.g. erectile difficulties or inability to bottom, in spite of willingness to do so, in anal sex in gay men), or automatic loss of ability to make even small gestures of same-gender intimacy when in public places (e.g. holding hands). Attunement to the client's embodied experience allows us to hypothesise about the extent to which the client's realm has been invaded by external oppression. In my experience, the more pervasive the oppression, the more embodied the symptoms in the client.

Sometimes the supervisee and/or supervisor get stuck in this cell. Excessive focus on the client's GSRD identity, without taking cognisance of the relational and contextual factors typical of cells 2, 3, 6, and 9, may be a sign of GSRD-targeted oppression. Especially if various events in the client's life, adversities, in particular, are understood as sole consequences of the client's GSRD identity.

- Cell 2: Client x Other; the clients' GSRD identities emerge at the cross-roads of biology and important life relationships. In this cell, the client's relational history of gender and sexuality is explored. Past and present client's relationships are a matter of inquiry here, with a special focus on their supportive potential. Who supported/supports the client as a GSRD person? What kind of support was/is it? If the client faced/faces a lack of support, what was/is their experience (someone's hatred or indifference towards them, homelessness, or loneliness)?

  What is more, being supported or not as a GSRD person over a lifetime must have shaped/must shape the client's endured relational themes. For instance, in my experience, the way the client's non-stereotypical gender behaviours were received by others frequently had a significant impact on the client's future sense of safety, adequacy, and shame in relationships. Importantly, it may also be hypothesised that the endured relational themes thus shaped may in turn influence the development of a GSRD identity in the client. For example, an adolescent cis-girl interested emotionally and sexually in other girls, when confronted with rage and love withdrawal from parents, may delay the development of her lesbian identity.

- Cell 3: Client x Situation; in this cell, the GSRD client's wider context is considered, especially their family and culture of origin. Above all, family messages – also transgenerational ones – on gender roles, sexual identity, sexual practices, forms of romantic and sexual relationships, and parenthood may significantly influence the client's understanding of "a proper life". In turn, it may potentially slow down or even arrest the process of a GSRD identity formation and make the client's personal life a struggle. For instance, a more egalitarian division of everyday duties and sex roles may be a complicated task in a relationship of two men, both coming from families with a rather rigid understanding of gender roles.

Moreover, the prism of dominant culture enables recognition of additional layers of the client's situation. Heteronormativity, with its homo-, bi-, trans-, and sexphobia, patriarchy, and misogyny, set harmful restrictions on GSRD psychological development and everyday life opportunities. For instance, depending on the specific socio-political conditions in a given country, gay men may be referred to conversion "therapist", convicted of an offence of "homosexual intercourse", or on the contrary – enabled to get married and become parents. This cell is the obvious one to discuss important intersections between the client's GSRD identity and other personal and contextual factors such as gender, age, disabilities, religion or spirituality, ethnic origin, financial resources, education, and social class. For example, a transgender person living in a village amongst a small religious community and being religious themselves will have different opportunities when it comes to coming-out, transition, or searching for a partner, in comparison to their city counterpart.

Significantly, GSRD-targeted oppressive attitudes on any part of the supervisory dyad will likely thwart crucial considerations typical of this cell. Discussing the oppressive environment requires unconditional acknowledgement of oppression being a fact.

- Cell 4: Supervisee x Self; this cell focuses on the supervisee's strengths and vulnerabilities in regard to discussing GSRD topics with the client. For example: Do they ask *all* clients about gender and sexual identity? Do they ask clients in same-gender relationships about sex life? Are they ready to discuss transition steps with transgender clients? Do they understand the heterogeneity of the asexual community? What is the strength or vulnerability of the supervisee that will sometimes depend mostly on their psychological and sexological knowledge? Which psychotherapeutic theory is implemented? Is it heteronormative by definition (e.g. classical psychoanalytic theory, some developmental character theories of psychodynamic origin)? Did the supervisee have specialist training in GSRD issues? However, also their personal history and resulting emotional capability, prejudices, and stereotypes are crucial, for instance, the supervisee reacting with overwhelming shame when confronted with sex issues, or the one assuming common heterosexuality or searching for "true homosexuality or transsexuality" may be a challenge for various groups of GSRD clients.

    Furthermore, this cell holds the space for a dialogue around the supervisee's GSRD identity. Is the supervisee a GSRD person themselves? If yes, what point of the GSRD identity process are they at? What are their self-supports considering being a GSRD professional? Answers to these questions will give the supervisor key information about possible effects (above all, potential harm) of the supervisee's internalised oppression on their clinical work with GSRD clients.

- Cell 5: Supervisee x Other; this cell directs attention to the "between" the supervisee and client. Such co-emergent phenomena may cover multiple aspects of contact. First of all, it is explored what is being imported from there-and-then to here-and-now of the relational field between the supervisee and client. This "bringing in" may concern both parts. The imported material may, for example, relate to the specific personal experiences and narratives about gender identity formation or sexuality development. For instance, a gay client (of any gender) shamed because of their gayness in the past, may expect shaming from the supervisee. On the other hand, the supervisee – laughed at and called "a faggot" at school for being a gender non-conforming boy – may feel anger towards their gay male client. Noteworthily, if the supervisee is a GSRD person themselves, with a life history similar to the client's, space for inclusion as well as the possibility of confluence on the supervisee's side arise. The first case will probably result in empathy for the client and a better understanding of them. The second will prevent the supervisee from perceiving the client as separate and different. For example, a transgender supervisee may find themselves really similar to their transgender client: coming out and transition narratives gave an effect of "sitting in front of a mirror". This unspoken and intuitive sense of connection with the client may paradoxically create a barrier to embrace the client as a whole human being, with everything that makes them different from the supervisee.

Further, in this cell, the client's and/or supervisee's disclosure of a GSRD identity is considered. Does the supervisee make a room for the client's coming out, or do they unspeakably solidify the social rule of staying silent about non-heteronormativity of any kind? The latter can result from, inter alia, the supervisee's withdrawal from any interest in the client's gender and sexuality issues. Additionally, if the supervisee is a GSRD person: Should they come out to the client, and if "yes" – then when? Answering these questions requires theoretical as well as clinical consideration.

This cell may also open exploration of romantic feelings and sexual attraction within a therapeutic relationship. Are the supervisee and supervisor ready to talk about, for instance, same-gender attraction in the therapeutic dyad? Do they have words for it? If, inauspiciously, the answer is "no", then – what is the reason for it?

From the thorough elaboration of the therapeutic relationship in supervision, the supervisee's GSRD-affirmative strategies and interventions in therapy emerge. Once again, not only are the supervisee's emotional availability and clinical expertise important, but also their practical knowledge. Frequently, it is more than useful to know the local GSRD communities, be able to refer to the nearest support groups for GSRD people, indicate medical centres prescribing PrEP, or understand how dating apps work.

- Cell 6: Supervisee x Situation; in this cell, the wider context of the client–supervisee relationship is considered. Taking the heteronormativity of a dominant culture into account, it is indispensable to be aware of ethical codes, guidelines, and position statements that bind the supervisee and secure the psychological safety of GSRD clients. A good example of such legal documents are existing in some countries' memoranda or resolutions which put a ban on so-called "conversion therapies". Professional ethics may be a starting point for a discussion on the therapeutic contract's details. For instance: does the supervisee want to contract for the conversion of one's sexual orientation, even though it is commonly regarded as unscientific, unethical and harmful? Does the supervisee combine roles of the therapist and diagnosing psychologist with transgender clients going through the gate-keeping procedure of gender transition? In my opinion, this roles mixing does not support therapy. If the supervisee works for an organisation, then organisational policies and internal procedures are of importance, for they may influence support services and the psychological well-being of GSRD clients.

  This cell explores also the supervisee's educational opportunities regarding GSRD issues in psychotherapy. Unfortunately, GSRD topics are frequently lacking from the general psychotherapy education programmes. In such a situation, the only way to improve qualifications is to attend specialised trainings, workshops, and supervision.

- Cell 7: Supervisor x Self; as it was with the Self dimension of the supervisee in Cell 4, in this cell the supervisor's strengths and vulnerabilities, when it comes to GSRD topics, are explored. Noteworthy, internalised supervisors – these echoes of the supervisor's past learning – may be important as models of attitudes towards GSRD in psychotherapy. Detailed characteristics of a GSRD-affirmative supervisor will be presented in the following section.

- Cell 8: Supervisor x Other; parallel processes are in focus in this cell. The supervisee brings in themselves the client's self to supervision (S. Denham-Vaughan, personal communication, 23 April 2021). This way what happens emotionally between the supervisee and client can be recaptured in the supervisory relationship. If noticed, this repeated situation can be analysed, providing important insights about the therapeutic process. For example, a supervisee working with a strongly homophobic gay client presents homophobic stereotypes during a supervisory consultation. This parallelism should be pointed out by the supervisor. However, such a scenario seems likely only under the condition of the supervisor's own readiness and efforts to confront their own homophobia (Cell 7).

- Cell 9: Supervisor x Situation; codes of ethics, position statements, and resolutions securing rights and psychological well-being of GSRD clients are important in this cell. In the case of clinical supervision delivered for supervisees working in organisations, also organisational policies and internal procedures should be scrutinised to protect the GSRD-affirmative stance.

The RMM's cells adapted in the GSRD-affirmative manner create a useful supervisory tool. The model's utility in GSRD-affirmative supervision will be illustrated with a fictitious clinical vignette.

A cis-male supervisee (45 years old), identifying himself as heterosexual (Cell 4), brings to supervision a dilemma from work with a cis-female client (54 years old), also identifying as heterosexual (Cell 1). The supervisor is a 65-year-old heterosexual and cis-female psychotherapist (Cell 7).

The client wants to explore her sex-related relationship issues. She says she is not able to understand her disinterest and inertia about sex. On one hand, she feels deficient as a woman, but on the other, she would not say she needs to be different. The client realises that she does not remember a time in her life when she missed having sex. She is a mother of two adult sons from the first marriage, and she points out that having children is the only beautiful and meaningful thing in her life that has resulted from sex (Cell 1). She was married twice, and divorced once again half a year ago. Both times she hoped that sex life would be more bearable, but it was not. As it was with her first husband, also the second one said he was not able to continue the relationship due to the lack of sex. She says that husbands left her with an explicit message she was the problem in the relationship. It is known from the client's sexual history that she was sexually abused as a teenager. Her then boyfriend, her first sexual partner (an 18-year-old) attempted to rape her when she was 17 years old (Cell 2). Moreover, the client comes from a rather traditional, Christian family with stereotyped perspective on woman's role as a wife, mother, and husband's support. She says it is not the first time she has seen a psychotherapist. The client had searched for help with sex-related issues in the past. However, she recollects the uselessness of the approach aimed at restoring her desire and willingness to have sex. It is clear that she was seen by professionals only through the lens of the Western assumptions about sex and sexuality. In a socio-cultural context where imperishable sexual desire is claimed to be a sexological and psychological norm, she was diagnosed with too low sexual desire levels and sexual aversion – both supposed to be related to the past sexual trauma (Cell 3).

The supervisee reports he has become stuck in his work with the client (Cell 5). He is married (Cell 4). Despite being quite open-minded, as he claims, he admits that his view of marriage and gender roles is rather traditional. For him, having sex is a natural and obvious consequence of feeling attracted to somebody or staying in a relationship. He was also trained in medical sexology, which strengthens his propensity to medicalise cultural phenomena, e.g. sexual exchange in couples.

A complete or temporary lack of sexual desire on either side of a dyad is to him a sign of somatic or relationship difficulties to be solved (Cell 6).

The supervisee recognises how challenging it is for him to understand the client differently than having a sexual disorder related to sexual trauma from her teenage years (Cell 5). The supervisor is an older woman and a feminist-informed systemic psychotherapist (Cell 7). As a result of her intellectual and past activism engagement in socio-cultural domain, she has a wider understanding of patriarchy and how a male-dominated perspective has influenced conceptualisation of women's sex lives and sexuality (Cell 9). She asks the supervisee about feelings. What are the client's feelings while presenting herself to the supervisee, a male psychotherapist (Cell 5)? What are the supervisee's feelings talking to the supervisor about his relationship with the client (Cell 8)? The supervisee instantly mentions shame. The client says a lot about how ashamed she feels in front of the supervisee because of her lack of interest in sex and disappointment she brought into her marriages (Cell 5). Interestingly, the supervisee reports also a parallel process with the supervisor. He talks about his own shame in front of the supervisor – a female psychotherapist. He reflects on his own shame around his helplessness and not being able to thoroughly understand and empathise with the female client's narrative on sex (Cell 8). It results with the supervisor's comment on the client's aspect that has never been fully acknowledged in psychotherapy, but was always a subject of reparative attempts from previous professionals: the client's lack of interest in sex. This absence of acceptance and validity confirmation has led to shame in the client's field, affecting the client herself and the supervisee as well. The supervisee is advised to look into affirmative psychotherapeutic narratives on asexuality. He is also prompted to propose this new label to the client; not necessarily to instantly identify with, but to equip her with a new positive tool that brings novel identity possibilities, fresh knowledge encouraging deeper self-understanding, a large community and sense of belonging, and above all validity as a human being. The supervisor then focuses the supervisee's attention on how an emotional bond and closeness are not identical to sexual attraction and do not have to be dependent on sexual acts (Cell 8 translating directly into intervention in Cell 5). The supervisor's perspective brings hope to the supervisee, supports his engagement in the therapeutic process, and reduces his own shame (Cell 8).

It is clear from the vignette how a supervision topic emerged among "the figure cells" (4, 5, 7, 8) from the ground shaped by Cells 1, 2, 3, 6, and 9. Supervisory work started with a dilemma in Cell 5 and finished with a suggestion of how to proceed in the therapeutic relationship (again Cell 5). The suggestion was a co-emergent result of working through the relationships between: (1) the supervisee and client, (2) the supervisee and supervisor, and (3) the client, supervisee, and supervisor, and their wider personal and/or professional contexts.

GSRD-affirmative supervisor

The supervisor's professional practice and theoretical consideration are reference points for supervisees, especially those still in training. It puts the responsibility on the supervisor. Specific areas of inquiry are listed next. They are a compilation of proposed supervisor's tasks and attitudes that support their GSRD-affirmative supervisory practice. According to my experience, a GSRD-affirmative supervisor should:

a) Be able to refer to the latest and cutting-edge research and knowledge on gender, sexuality, and relationship issues in psychotherapy and supervision.
b) Understand the social context of various GSRD identities.
c) Make a personalised diagnosis of difficulties brought by GSRD clients and supervisees, taking intersectionality into account.
d) Be aware of their own cis-het-mononormative assumptions and behaviours.
e) Be aware of their own homo-, bi-, transphobia, and heterosexism.
f) Be aware of their own gender stereotype beliefs.
g) Be aware of various aspects of their own gender identity and roles, and sexuality.

The list allows to distinguish two separate areas of a GSRD-affirmative supervisor's professional development: (1) gaining specialist knowledge (a–c) and (2) building up wider self-understanding (d–g). The area of knowledge can be advanced through training, supervision, reading, films, and being part of the GSRD community – also as an ally. The area of self-understanding can grow in psychotherapy, regular re-assessment of one's own attitudes towards gender, sexuality, and different forms of sexual and/or romantic relationships, and in sex education. Furthermore, in my opinion, attending anti-discrimination training is also required for a GSRD-affirmative supervisor's development. Exclusively through knowing their own discriminatory stance against not only a given gender or sexuality but also religion, spirituality, age, disability, social class, etc., will the supervisor be able to look at the client through the intersectionality prism. Importantly, the supervisor's self-awareness cannot be replaced by their – even excellent – general knowledge on gender, sexual, and relationship diversity. Extraordinary factual knowledge may become useless when blended with unconscious incompetence in the form of homo-, bi-, trans-, sexphobia, or misogyny.

Summary

The RMM model accentuates the significance of the ground conditions that pre-configure what becomes figural in supervision. In GSRD-affirmative supervision, the ground conditions are important in a unique way. Only the supervisory focus on the framing cells 1, 2, 3, 6, and 9 can fully reveal oppression mechanisms and enables acknowledgement of GSRD people as a group of clients with special needs in therapy. The RMM's cells can be discussed individually, but they are actually interconnected. A smooth supervisory work, supportive of the client's integration, requires access to all cells. To make it possible, the supervisor should be aware of and professionally trained in working with all the RMM's cells (Chidiac et al., 2017). In terms of GSRD-affirmative supervision, it means that additional and specific GSRD-knowledgeable expertise is needed on the supervisor's side.

References

Aylward, J. (2018). *The Anarchy of Gestalt Therapy: A Proposal for Radical Practice*. Peregian Beach, Australia: Ravenwood Press.

Bąk, D. (2021). Psychotherapy in the shadow of shame: The Polish experience of institutionalized homo-, bi-, and transphobia. *The Jung Journal: Culture & Psyche, 15*(4), 7–20.

Baumann, P. (2007). Persons, human beings, and respect. *Polish Journal of Philosophy, 1*(2), 5–17.

Caroll, M., & Gilbert, M. C. (2011). *On Being a Supervisee: Creating Learning Partnerships* (3rd ed.). Kew, Australia: PsychOz Publications.

Chidiac, M.-A., Denham-Vaughan, S., & Osborne, L. (2017). The relational matrix model of supervision: Context, framing and inter-connection. *British Gestalt Journal, 28*(2), 21–30.

Clark-Polner, E., & Clark, M. S. (2014). Understanding and accounting for relational context is critical for social sciences. *Frontiers in Human Neuroscience, 8*, 1–14. Retrieved July 31, 2021, from www.ncbi.nlm.nih.gov/pmc/articles/PMC3971189/pdf/fnhum-08-00127.pdf

Denham-Vaughan, S., & Chidiac, M.-A. (2013). SOS: A relational orientation towards social inclusion. *Mental Health and Social Inclusion, 17*(2), 100–107.

Gilbert, M. C., & Evans, K. (2000). *Psychotherapy Supervision: An Integrative Relational Approach to Psychotherapy Supervision*. Buckingham: Open University Press.

Hawkins, P., & Shohet, R. (1989). *Supervision in the Helping Professions*. Buckingham: Open University Press.

Hawkins, P., & Shohet, R. (2006). *Supervision in the Helping Professions* (3rd ed.). Maidenhead: Open University Press.

Hayes, S. C. (2004). Acceptance and commitment therapy, relational frame theory, and the third wave of behavioral and cognitive therapies. *Behavior Therapy, 35*(4), 639–665.

Jacobs, L. (2004). Ethics of context and field: The practices of care, inclusion and openness to dialogue. In R. G. Lee (Ed.), *The Voices of Connection: A Relational Approach to Ethics* (1st ed., pp. 35–55). Hillsdale, NY: GestaltPress/The Analytic Press.

Jacobs, L. (2009). Relationality: Foundational assumptions. In D. Ullman & G. Wheeler (Eds.), *CoCreating the Field: Intention and Practice in the Age of Complexity* (1st ed., pp. 41–66). Santa Cruz, CA: GestaltPress.

Jacobs, L. (2017a). Hopes, fears, and enduring relational themes. *British Gestalt Journal, 26*(1), 7–16.

Jacobs, L. (2017b). On dignity, a sense of dignity, and inspirational shame. *Psychoanalytic Inquiry, 37*(6), 380–394.

Jacobs, L., & Hycner, R. (Eds.). (2009). *Relational Approaches in Gestalt Therapy*. Santa Cruz, CA and Orleans, MA: GestaltPress.

Mizen, C. S., & Hook, J. (2020). Relational and affective neuroscience: A quiet revolution in psychiatric and psychotherapeutic practice. *BJPsych Advances, 26*(Special Issue 6), 356–366.

Resnick, R. F., & Estrup, L. (2000). Supervision. A collaborative endeavor. *Gestalt Review*, *4*(2), 121–137.

Safran, J. D., & Kraus, J. (2015). Relational techniques in a cognitive-behavioral therapy context: "It's bigger than the both of us". In N. C. Thoma & D. McKay (Eds.), *Working with Emotion in Cognitive-Behavioral Therapy: Techniques for Clinical Practice* (1st ed., pp. 333–55). New York, NY: The Guilford Press.

Stolorow, R. D., Atwood, G. E., & Brandchaft, B. (1994). *The Intersubjective Perspective*. Northvale, NJ: Jason Aronson.

Wachtel, P. L. (2010). *Relational Theory and the Practice of Psychotherapy*. New York: The Guilford Press.

Chapter 13

Living and working within our communities

Dominic Davies

Introduction

This chapter mainly aims at GSRD-identified therapists who often feel they are working on the edges of the profession, trying to ride the boundary (Gabriel, 2005) between living and working within their community and navigating ethical dilemmas using heteronormative and mononormative lenses to help them reflect on the challenges. More specifically, I'm seeking to address those therapists who are actively dating and socialising within the LGBTQIA+ communities.

Due to the complexity of the subject and trying to manage the constraints of chapter length, I shall be making several assumptions and asking the reader to find their ethical boundaries in the scenarios I present. Rehearsing one's ethical thinking is likely to make for a therapist who can be responsive rather than paralysed with fear when similar boundary issues arise in their own lives.

I will explore how personal and professional, ethical boundaries may become blurred when therapists are actively involved in the LGBTQIA+ communities. I will also offer examples of how these boundary dilemmas might play out in real life. I hope that by the end of this chapter, readers will better understand how to approach these matters and some frameworks and tools for managing them.

Assumption one: the therapist is out to their GSRD clients

Therapist self-disclosure has been a matter of much controversy over the four decades I've been practising as a therapist. It was thought to interfere with therapeutic neutrality and the now antiquated concept of the 'blank screen' required by psychoanalytic practitioners to allow the development of a transference-based relationship. "The doctor should be opaque to his patients and, like a mirror, should show them nothing but what is shown to him" (Freud, 1912, pp. 117–118). Nowadays, this is heavily contested thinking as the therapist constantly discloses information about themselves, in terms of their gender, class, age, clothing, location, accent, body size and what they choose to respond to and what they remain silent about.

DOI: 10.4324/9781003260561-14

I can think of only very few examples where it's ethically and clinically justifiable that the therapist would hide their sexuality. The first example is if the therapist lives in a country where homosexuality is illegal, they could risk arrest. The second is if the therapist works in forensic settings where personal information can be used to manipulate staff members. In all other cases, I think that it's possible to be selectively out to clients and colleagues, and I would strongly argue that it's in the interests of the client, the therapeutic relationship and the therapist to be open. I am also sure there would be colleagues in those settings who have selectively disclosed. However, if there are sound clinical or personal safety reasons not to tell, then I think the therapist could address the client's motivation for asking the question. This should be done with great care and respect to avoid a therapeutic rupture. Motivations for knowing something personal are often the client's attempt to meet Roger's first Condition, that of *Psychological Contact* (Davies & Aykroyd, 2002). It could also be an attempt to assess your cultural competence and experience in working with GSRD-specific issues.

If, on the other hand, the therapist is still coming to terms with their own sexuality, they should consider if they are feeling integrated enough to take this client on and ensure an experienced GSRD-informed supervisor supervises their work to regularly monitor for unintended counter-transferential reactions, much as one might after a significant personal bereavement. Personal therapy would also be highly recommended.

New York psychoanalyst Jack Drescher maintains: "Gay therapists who live closeted, professional lives have a particular need *to* hide. They also experience their own homosexuality as something secretive and shameful" (Drescher, 1998, p. 228).

Over the decades, we have moved from 'Thou Shalt Not' to self-disclosure, which can be highly beneficial for developing the therapeutic relationship (Jeffery & Tweed, 2015) when done selectively and in the client's service. For readers who want to know more about the matter, I recommend you read Satterly (2006), Harris, (2015) and Danzer (2019).

Nowadays, GSRD therapists are often out by implication – they might mention they work with GSRD or LGBTQIA+ clients on their websites without directly mentioning their identifications. Clients then might assume the therapist has some direct knowledge of their worlds. This isn't to say all GSRD therapists are familiar with all aspects of a particular identity/community. Still, in my experience, even heterosexual, married and monogamous therapists who work with GSRD clients usually do so because they have some identification with the GSRD spectrum; perhaps a kink identification, an unexpressed bisexual orientation, or possibly parenting a queer child, for example. To paraphrase Avenue Q, "We're all a little bit GSRD!"

The situation is more complicated if one works within an organisation and is assumed to be cisgender-heterosexual and monogamous. One will hopefully be working in a country where you have equal and anti-discrimination employment rights and can't be fired for being GSRD. I would recommend you come out to at least some of your colleagues as a source of support, but I would also encourage you to be out to clients by inference if not directly. Have some queer iconography and symbolism in your office, some queer therapy textbooks on your desk or bookshelves, a rainbow flag/badge, etc. Coming out to clients needn't be a 'big deal' and intruding on their own story; it can more naturally occur by implication as most clients will be scanning for signs of safety and queerness. Regardless of whether you are out to your clients or not, you will still need to have robustly considered how you will manage the potential of meeting your clients outside of the therapy room.

Assumption two: the therapist is honest, ethical, and minded to work in the best interests of the client/patient

I prefer to assume an optimistic and positivistic view of therapists. Whilst the initial training for many therapists in working with GSRD clients is woefully inadequate, I would prefer to take the view that therapists are not being deliberately incompetent. A more plausible explanation is that they may be naive to the impact that cisgenderism, heteronormativity and mononormativity have had on them and their world views and that they've, in large, been poorly served by the training programmes that fail to adequately prepare them for the demands of specialist work with a traumatised, minority population. Therapists frequently do not know what they do not know and are often unaware of what it takes to work well with GSRD clients. I often hear the epithet that 'people are people, and we're all the same underneath.' I agree with this statement, but it's highly reductionist to deny the significant differences between cisgender and trans folks and heterosexuals and queers and a major microaggression to deny the impact of minority stress. Therapists need training in both cultural sensitivity and cultural humility (Tervalon & Murray-Garcia, 1998; Stubbe, 2020) to be effective with GSRD clients (Davies & Neves, 2023).

Assumption three: therapists have a right to social, sexual and relational lives and participate fully in their community's social and political activities

As therapists, we have ethical and moral obligations to practise self-care, to keep a balance between mind, body and, if one believes in such things, our spirit or soul. We know from resilience research that connection to the LGBTQIA+ communities is a protective factor in acting as an antidote to endemic heteronormativity and minority stress (Meyer, 2015). Time spent with our communities or tribes can be very restorative. Engaging with queer social and cultural events and watching LGBTQIA+ TV films and series can create a sense of belonging and identity formation. I'm aware some of my colleagues live in Queer-hostile environments, and I urge you to find support for your identity and lives online if there is little locally safe or developed.

We should not rely on our queer clients as our only connection to the queer community, living vicariously through their adventures. But I've heard many therapists say they're afraid of accessing the queer community for fear of running into clients, so they withdraw from actively participating. I don't think this is a healthy or safe practice for therapists or their work with GSRD clients.

Therapists need to pay attention to the world of our intimate relationships. I've met many single therapists who long to be in intimate relationships and spend their lives helping clients with their relationship issues. Still, their sexual and relational worlds are a desert. I think we need to be able to do more than talk the walk. We owe ourselves and our clients to put some energy into our social and sexual lives. Whilst many people find certain dating apps to be toxic environments (Pachankis et al., 2020), there are many ways in which we can find to connect socially (and sexually if that's desired) with our communities.

The notion that monogamy is the only way to have a successful and fulfilling relationship is outdated and, as we've seen throughout this book, simply not true. For many, monogamy isn't the right fit – and that's perfectly okay. For others, their monogamous relationship might end, and they find themselves back out in the dating pool with other single and CNM therapists, mixing in the same crowd and maybe on the same apps as their clients. We need to find ways to manage this better.

Assumption four: sexual contact between therapist and client is unethical and inappropriate

There is one sub-branch of our profession where these rules might not be inviolable. This might be in the case of trained somatic sexologists, sexological bodyworkers and sexual surrogates, whose work may involve intimate touch under very particular circumstances. In the first two of those professions, it might involve one-way touch using gloves for any intimate body contact. For the counselling, psychotherapy, psychosexual and relationship therapy professions, sexualised touch violates the trust placed in us by all our clients, colleagues and professional membership bodies. Therapists need to be trained and able to work therapeutically with erotic energies and the feelings of love and desire that can naturally arise in psychotherapy (Shlien, 1984). I can think of no ethical justification for violating this universal rule, and considerable work has been done to understand the damage to clients where their therapist has engaged in sexual contact with them (Pope et al., 2005).

One might pause to consider what is meant by 'sexual contact.' This area is rooted in cis-het mononormative contexts. The writers of the Code of Ethics (BACP, 2018; COSRT, 2022; UKCP, 2019) probably understand this phrase means no sexual *touching and definitely no sexual intercourse*, but what about being dressed provocatively in the lounge area of a swingers club? What if the therapist and client are both in the same gay sauna, not interacting with each other but dressed in a towel on the same premises? How about the client walking in on the therapist giving a flogging to someone in a kink dungeon party? Might it be different if the client were to witness the therapist receiving a flogging? Is flogging even a sexual act? The codes aren't clear, and these are great topics to bring to an experienced GSRD-informed supervisor or to discuss with GSRD colleagues.

Assumption five: the therapist is likely to be single or non-monogamous

For this chapter, I want to hold in our minds the therapist who is not in a monogamous relationship but is either single or open to meeting and dating other people. First, I want to state that it's perfectly fine to be single and not want to date. There is often pressure to be dating or having lots of sex, which isn't helpful for aromantic and asexual therapists. There has been a longstanding heteronormative and mononormative assumption in our profession that therapists should be coupled in a 'committed relationship,' which I always feel is a code for being monogamous. Most people in Consensually Non-Monogamous relationships would also consider themselves in committed relationships. There is an expectation that we should avoid at all costs being in the same social spaces as our clients. When one considers the divorce rate for marriages and the frequency of extra-marital 'infidelity,' the expectation and pressure of lifelong monogamy are likely to be very shaming for many therapists of all sexualities.

Assumption six: dual and multiple relationships and boundary crossings are inevitable in working with minority communities where one is also a member

As with GPs and Clergy working in rural communities, GSRD-identified therapists are also highly likely to meet their fellow community members outside the consulting room even if they live in big cities, this may be a meeting about social and political issues, Pride events or in bars and clubs, at the gym or even in the case of queer parents, the school playground. It might also be in more sexualised spaces, kink dungeon playrooms, saunas, cruising grounds or intimate dinner parties with friends and ex-lovers. I believe we need to anticipate this happening, plan how we might manage it, and guide our clients on how we will be doing our best to preserve the therapeutic relationship and navigate our mutual paths within the community that sustains us.

I know from experience as a practice consultant that many therapists find it difficult to bring these boundary dilemmas to their cis-het supervisors, whom they fear won't understand the social contexts of their lives or who may judge them through mononormative perspectives. Let us start by introducing a case example to help illustrate some of the points we need to consider.

Case study

Jacob is a 42-year-old married gay man recently single after his husband of 20 years left him for a younger man. Jacob is a therapist working primarily from their home with the GSRD communities.

One of Jacob's roles in the relationship was maintaining their home life, cooking, shopping, etc. It meant he could work from home and see clients. When the relationship ended, and the flat was sold, Jacob was given a settlement, which meant leaving their home and local friends and moving further out of London, jeopardising his private practice.

Jacob believed he and Daniel were in a monogamous relationship. He met his husband when he was 22 and Daniel was 35. He moved in and settled into Daniel's flat. Five years later, they married, and everything felt very settled, Jacob thought he would be with Daniel forever. A decade ago, Jacob trained as a psychotherapist, and Daniel supported him in training by covering all the living costs as a couple and assisting with his course fees.

Jacob has remained in therapy and has been using that space to explore his rage and loss and work out how to move forwards. In the two decades he has been with Daniel, the dating world has changed significantly. Grindr and other geolocation smartphone apps didn't exist when he was single. Also, when he met Daniel, he'd only had a few short-term dating-type relationships. Jacob needs to navigate dating and is very worried about encountering clients online and in real life when he goes out to gay social spaces.

Jacob created a profile on Grindr and found no one wanted to chat with him as he wasn't comfortable sharing a photo of his face in case a client recognised him. Many of his clients knew he was gay, and he'd learned through supervision and dialogue with colleagues that selective self-disclosure was acceptable when in the client's interests. But he didn't feel comfortable 'announcing my sexual interests to everyone.'

Davies et al. (2016) undertook a brief survey into App use amongst gay male therapists and sexual health care workers ($N = 195$). Eighty-five per cent of the respondents had a Grindr profile. Forty-seven per cent of the respondents had a picture of their face and were clothed on their profile. Twenty-five per cent did not display a face or torso shot and would presumably send one after checking out who they were speaking with.

Jacob soon learned first-hand what his clients had reported to him in his therapy room, the toxic nature of the competitiveness, the rejection of gay men who were older and who didn't spend five days a week in the gym, the intracommunity gay minority stress, the 'shade' culture of put-downs and the search for high status, wealthy, and hung partners (Pachankis et al., 2020). He deleted Grindr.

Jacob went to hook up with someone who offered him mephedrone and GHB/GBL, two of the specific drugs used for chemsex (Stuart, 2016), and he had wild abandoned sex for 24 hours. They met again, and his lover suggested they get a couple more guys over the next time. Jacob had little sexual experience before meeting Daniel, and the drugs pressed the 'play' button on his adolescent psychosexual development. He found himself wanting to meet more people and have sex for longer and in more creative ways. Several months went by, and one weekend, Jacob turned up to a small chillout (a term for chemsex parties) of four guys and found one of his clients high on GHB. Jacob left immediately, grateful he hadn't taken anything himself. He was overcome with guilt and shame. After an emergency consultation with his supervisor, Jacob decided that the risks of group sex and chemsex were too much for him, and he stopped taking up such invitations.

At his next session and for a couple of further sessions, Jacob and his client discussed the impact of meeting outside the therapy room in a sexualised context. The client saw Jacob as someone with the same needs for sex and recreation; Jacob became a real person rather than simply a 'therapist.' The client did not have a problematic relationship with drug use, which wasn't the primary reason he consulted Jacob. There was no complicated history of trauma or sexual abuse. Jacob was able to help his client process the meaning of this out-of-session contact and, with the benefit of additional supervision sessions, work through this unusual boundary crossing. Had the situation been reversed, or in the case of a client with a different history, it would more likely have been a boundary violation and an entirely different outcome.

Whilst most codes of ethics warn of the dangers of dual and multiple relationships, within smaller communities (rural, recovery, or faith communities) they are accepted as inevitable. They are also unavoidable when the therapist identifies as GSRD and works with their community. Ofer Zur (2022) informs us that there are two types of boundary crossings.

> Boundary violations and boundary crossings in psychotherapy refer to any deviation from traditional, strict, 'only in the office,' emotionally distant forms of therapy. They mostly refer to issues of self-disclosure, length and place of sessions, physical touch, activities outside the office, gift exchange, social and other non-therapeutic contact and various forms of dual relationships. Basically, they may all be seen as a departure from the traditional psychoanalytic proceedings.
>
> (Zur, O Zur Institute)

Boundary violations are harmful to the therapeutic relationship, whereas boundary crossings are not and indeed can be beneficial.

One of the tasks Jacob's supervisor set him was to create a Professional Boundaries Statement which could be integrated into his therapy contract or sit alongside it as a separate document that he might selectively give to clients who overlap his social networks. He would share this document with his clients to guide them on how they might manage out-of-session contact in the various online and social settings that Jacob frequented. This would then be discussed early in the contracting stage of the work with a new client.

Writing a professional boundaries statement

Task one

- List all the dating apps you use. Note which ones you have a picture of your face on and if you've been explicit about what you're looking for.
- List all the Social Media apps you're on and consider how you will deal with friend requests and solicitations coming via social media.
- List the venues where you socialise and/or look for potential partners or where you might seek to find sex or even new friends.
- List your domestic arrangement, whom you share your living space with (partner(s), flatmates, family and how you might interact with people in that space; i.e. if you have an open relationship and your partner or flatmate unwittingly brings home a client, or if you are a parent and your children want playdates with a client's children).
- List all the organisations you might volunteer in and meet other people.

Task two

Consider how you will manage 'meeting' or having contact with a client in some of these settings. Which one seems most challenging for you?

(Think communal changing rooms, being 'under the influence' at a birthday celebration in a pub for your or a best friend's birthday, being messaged on a dating app, attending a workshop, community event or private party where your client is also a guest or your kids become friends with a client's family, etc. . . .).

Now write a series of guidelines for you and your clients on managing these situations ethically and preserving the therapeutic frame. This document is now your Professional Boundaries Statement.

Here are three examples of what a Professional Boundaries statement could look like. Used anonymously, with permission from graduates of our Diploma programme.

Example one: professional boundaries statement

This professional boundaries statement provides you and me with guidance and rules for the duration of our therapy work together. Boundaries are not barriers; they are meant to help you and me maintain a professional, confidential, and ethical relationship. They also allow for safe and authentic therapeutic work towards your therapy goals.

Sometimes you and I might have social connections other than through our therapy work, often referred to as 'multiple relationships.' Those multiple relationships are a common reality for practitioners working in 2SLGBTIQ+ communities and can involve social and digital spaces. If the potential for multiple relationships exists between you and me, it is important that we openly address those as part of the therapeutic process. This is important because openly discussing your and my experiences and knowledge within 2SLGBTIQ+ communities will allow us to explore and better understand how shared involvement in a 2SLGBTIQ+ community may affect the dynamics of your therapy. It also provides you with a choice and allows you to reflect critically on whether you feel comfortable working with me or not. At the same time, it also allows me to openly discuss with you if I have any concerns that might limit our ability to work together. In such a situation, we would discuss alternative ways of interacting with each other that would make therapy more permissible, or we could consider alternative treatment options, and I would help you access those options.

If you know of any shared social spaces between you and me, please raise them during our therapy sessions. The sheer fact of inhabiting overlapping social spaces (shared communities, shared volunteering or community participation, shared personal relationships) does not prevent us from having a therapeutic relationship. There are many ways in which therapists maintain professional boundaries while having multiple relationships with clients, as long as those are within the boundaries of the code of ethical conduct of the governing body for my therapy work. However, not disclosing knowledge about shared social spaces can harm our relationship and inadvertently become a boundary violation. I commit to addressing any potential overlaps in our social spaces if I become aware of them. I also commit to openly addressing any conflict of interest I might identify during our therapy process. Please address any potential shared places you might be aware of during our therapy session.

The dynamic, complex, and changeable use of social media means that a finite set of rules cannot meet professional safety in social media. What is required is a therapeutic approach, a way of thinking and reflecting on the impact of social media. In my practice, I will not knowingly connect with my clients outside of our agreed communication channels (i.e. typically e-mail, telephone or text message, as you prefer). If I am providing you with additional information relating to digital spaces (e.g. websites, apps, social media accounts), I commit to providing you with professional content relating to our therapeutic work only. I will not knowingly connect with you outside of these boundaries (e.g. Twitter, Facebook, recreational networking apps, etc.). In return, I expect that you do not attempt to connect with me outside of our agreed communication channels unless we have explicitly discussed this in our therapy sessions and have worked through our shared understanding of the impact and indication for any exemptions. Should either of us unknowingly and unintentionally realize that these rules were violated, it is of utmost importance that we discuss this during therapy and find ways of resolving any such situation.

Please bring any questions or thoughts you might have about this professional boundaries statement to our next therapy session.

Example two: professional boundaries statement – things I would add to my contract

Being visible in the community

I hold to the tenet generally applicable in the therapy community around the client–therapist relationship that no dual relationships are allowed, romantic or otherwise. I also hold my work to standard moral principles that underlie counselling, particularly non-maleficence and justice, meaning what would cause the least harm and what would be fairest for us in this relationship. I would like to outline, however, some grey areas around this, as we may encounter each other outside of the therapy room, historically, in the present, or in the future

1.   Physical spaces

As queer communities are somewhat smaller than hetero communities, there is an increased likelihood that our paths may cross outside of the therapy room. And as a queer therapist myself, it is an important part of my identity to access the various scenes here in Berlin. I list some examples below, these lists not being exhaustive, but just to give you an idea:

- Queer parties, e.g. Same Bitches, Riot, Transmission.
- Queer venues (clubs, bars, museums), e.g. Schwuz, Berghain, Südblock, Roses, Rauschgold, Schwules Museum, Ficken3000.
- Queer festivals/outdoor spaces, e.g. Whole Festival, Hasenheide, FKK (naked) areas which are common around most Berlin lakes and some parks.
- Queer events: film festivals, art shows.
- Queer collectives: the Village, Karada house.
- Queer gatherings: protests, vigils, marches.

Normally, I contract with new clients if we see each other out and about (at any of the above, for example). Notwithstanding my Confidentiality statement written earlier in this working contract, I would not acknowledge you should I see you. Still, you are welcome to acknowledge me (a nod, a smile, a hello) if you wish, and I will respond in kind. Of course, you can choose not to acknowledge me, which is fine.

And if we are still in therapy together, as part of my commitment to the boundaries of our therapeutic relationship, I would like to invite a reflection of the sighting of each other after the event (next session) so that we can process anything that may have come up for you.

Should we no longer be in therapy together, obviously I can't check in with you, but we can review this at the end of our treatment together.

Finally, regarding queer club venues, you may see me dancing half naked, and we can talk about this in the first session, addressing what comes up for both of us (and at a later date if this is applicable).

2. *Sexualised spaces*

I am not currently attending Play, Chill Out or Kink/BDSM parties here in Berlin. This also pertains to Dark Room spaces, some of which are attached to bars and are present in most queer parties. Additionally, I'm not currently attending outdoor cruising spaces in Berlin (Hasenheide, Tiergarten, for example).

However, I do attend FKK (naked) areas in the summertime now and again, e.g. Karlsdorfer See and Krumme Lanke, so we can negotiate in the first session what this might be like for both of us, should this apply to you (and also at a later date if this is applicable).

3. *Virtual spaces*

I can be on the following apps:

- Grindr.
- Tinder.
- Planet Romeo.
- OK Cupid.
- Feeld.

It is usually my policy, as a right to privacy, that if I see a client on an app (particularly Grindr), I will block them. Let me know how you might feel about this. And as per my statement above regarding contact out of session, if you do message me on any of these apps, I will not respond but will talk about it with you in the next session following the contact. If we have ended therapy, I would ask you to remember this contract, as we will not be able to resolve anything that comes up for you if you have contacted me on these apps.

4. *Past, current and future us*

Suppose it becomes apparent, during the initial stages of our therapy, that I know with some degree of intimacy or regularity people that are close to you (current lover, an ex, close friend, for example). In that case, I will bring this into the room. We may decide that this duality is manageable in the context of this therapeutic relationship (possibly with further boundaries). However, we will likely have to end our relationship, and I can refer you to another therapist.

Per my statement above regarding Dual Relationships, we will not be able to enter into a romantic relationship or friendship in the future once we have started a therapeutic relationship.

And as this is a working contract for both of us, I would invite any feedback, criticism, or reflection on any of the above as part of an ongoing contracting process in this therapeutic relationship.

Example three: professional boundaries agreement for polyam and/or kinky clients

This agreement does not replace or negate any of the boundaries established through our pre-existing contract, which establishes boundaries according to standard professional guidelines. The pre-existing contract states that you have a right to confidentiality, that I am bound to both ethically and by law and that I can only break this if there is a risk of immediate, significant, and sustained harm to yourself or another person. It also states that if we meet in public, to maintain your confidentiality, I will only greet you if you greet me first.

In some LGBTQ+ affirmative contexts where we may meet, e.g., LGBTQ+ oriented sports clubs or bars, the pre-existing contract will generally suffice as although these are LGBTQ+ affirmative spaces, they are not centred explicitly around sexual or kink/BDSM-related activities.

This statement is intended to enhance our understanding of our already established boundaries so that they can cover spaces explicitly centred around sex/kink/BDSM as well. My intention in us each agreeing to the boundaries in this statement is that we will be able to work together without destabilising our therapeutic relationship or compromising our freedom to participate in these spaces and communities.

I greatly value my life experience within queer, polyam and kinky communities and how this experience informs my ability to work with clients whose therapy may focus on navigating identities, desires and relationship practise related to these same aspects of experience/identity.

Simultaneously, I am aware of unique situations we may be required to navigate as part of sharing subcultural spaces in this manner. Specifically, publicly dating and socialising in environments shared with my clients means we are more likely to witness or learn about each other's erotic or relationship practices. Therefore, this statement lays out some boundaries I expect myself and my clients to maintain to manage these situations.

Whilst I am involved in Polyamorous relationships and kink/BDSM scenes where we may crossover, this managed and negotiated form of disclosure feels appropriate and preferable to an accidental crossing of boundaries, which could have happened were this disclosure not made via this agreement.

Kink/BDSM Boundaries

• If we intend to be in a public sex and/or public kink/BDSM play space, if either one of us knows the other will be in the same space beforehand, we agree to alert the other of this fact and discuss beforehand an etiquette specific to the space, that we will each follow.

In all cases, we agree:

• Not to engage in any kind of sexual/kink-related activity with each other.

- Not to watch or listen to each other's sexual or 'play' activities.
- Furthermore, we agree to do what we can to prevent finding out about the other person's activities by talking to other people who may have engaged in or witnessed such activities.
- If we find each other's profiles on dating, kink or hook-up apps, or any social media associated with public sex/play spaces, we agree not to read them or look at media posted on them.
- I have taken the decision not to engage in any social media which are specifically for the purpose of posting nudes or 'thirst traps' (whether anonymously or otherwise) so as to avoid potentially encroaching on client's boundaries.
- In addition, we could make an agreement that if we ever do find ourselves in a public sex/play space where we are unsure how to navigate boundaries, whilst at the venue we can contact each other via text in order to arrange how to navigate this discreetly. This being the case you can text me on my work mobile. This is an option but is not obligatory – please do let me know what you would feel comfortable with.
- If we are in sex/kink affirmative space where play or sex doesn't happen, e.g., a munch, we will follow the same principle shared in the contract, i.e. I only say hello if you greet me first and if we do speak, I will not say anything that might disclose the fact you are my client or refer to the content of our therapy sessions.
- Additionally, you may choose to out yourself as my client or break your own confidentiality. Whilst I would not encourage this, this would be your prerogative.

Polyam Boundaries

- If, in the context of being in non-monogamous relationships, we feel that the professional boundaries of our relationship might be compromised because of who we are dating or who our partners are dating etc., we will agree to inform each other and negotiate how to respond to the situation on a case by case basis.

Ethical frameworks

It's up to you whether you selectively share your statement with clients where you share social spaces or routinely give it to all your GSRD clients, but I would highly recommend you prepare such a statement and discuss it with your supervisor.

Let us now turn to apply ourselves to working on some ethical dilemmas. I believe the more one applies oneself to consider scenarios where boundary crossings occur, the more adept one can become at managing these with care, compassion and ethical integrity.

There are several models of ethical decision-making around boundaries (Gabriel & Davies, 2000; Forester-Miller & Davis, 2016; Lazarus & Zur, 2002;

Pope & Vasquez, 2016). I will draw upon the model developed by Lynne Gabriel, presented in a couple of different incarnations, not least the chapter she and I wrote in Pink Therapy vol 3 (Gabriel & Davies, 2000); it will hopefully be familiar to many readers and embrace many alternative models' points.

Process model for ethical problem solving and decision making

This is the overarching framework for dealing with ethical dilemmas with the practical steps involved.

1   **Write a brief description of the problem or dilemma**.

This helps minimise confusion and is particularly helpful when discussing the situation with your supervisor or colleague.

2   **Whose problem or dilemma is it?**

- The therapists?
- The clients?
- Joint problem?
- Agency/organisation problem?

3   **Consider ethics, codes and guidelines**.

- Consider appropriate sources of guidance, e.g. your professional body's codes and guidelines.
- What actions are prohibited or required according to available ethics codes?
- What actions are required by law?

4   **Consider the moral principles underlying counselling/psychotherapy**.

- Beneficence: what will achieve the greatest good?
- Non-maleficence: what will cause the least harm?
- Justice: what will be the fairest for all parties involved?
- Respect for autonomy: what maximises opportunities for choice?
- Fidelity: what actions ensure the therapist remains faithful to the therapeutic relationship? Therapy is a *fiduciary* relationship; it is given in trust. Breaking the client's trust in the therapist constitutes a serious violation of the therapeutic relationship, and reparation and redemption of the alliance might not be possible.

5   **Identify possible courses of action**.

Brainstorm all possible courses of action. Depending upon the circumstances, this step will be carried out with the client, supervisor and counselling colleague's support and cooperation.

6   **Select the most appropriate course of action**.

Consider the preferred course of action from the following perspectives:

- *Universality*: could the chosen action be recommended to others? Would I condone it if undertaken by a colleague?
- *Publicity*: could I explain my chosen action to colleagues? Supervisor? Would I be willing to expose it to scrutiny in court, media or other public forums?
- *Justice*: would I take the same action with other clients? Would my decision have been the same if the client were well-known or influential? Different?

Answering *no* to any of these questions indicates a need to reconsider, preferably with your supervisor.

7   **Evaluate the outcome**.

Consider:

- Was the outcome as you hoped?
- Had you considered all relevant factors so that no new factors emerged?
- Would you do the same again in similar circumstances?

If you answered *no* to any of these questions, consider what you would do differently.

Working with dilemmas in dual relationships and overlapping connections

Stage 1: impact and containment

This stage requires immediate actions such as:

- Contain shock and impact of situation.
- Invoke stress/crisis management techniques.
- Contain any immediate 'fallout'/acting-out impulses.
- Invoke an 'internal supervisor.'
- Make contact with the client, acknowledge the situation.
- Seek agreement to discuss the situation at the next therapy session.
- Model healthy, appropriate behaviour.

Stage 2: containment and processing

This stage requires intermediate actions and acknowledging the situation at the next therapy session.

- Discuss with client issues of confidentiality, boundaries, overlapping connections and possible rehearsal of agreed actions should other situations arise.
- Address the client's reactions/responses to the situation.
- Address transference issues.
- Provide ongoing containment.
- Redeem the therapeutic alliance.
- Discuss countertransference reactions in supervision and personal therapy.

Stage 3: ongoing processing

This stage is about the longer-term effect of the dual relationship and overlapping connections.

- Explore transference and countertransference in personal therapy and supervision.
- Work with issues triggered by or linked to dual or multiple roles and relationships.
- Apply your ethical decision-making skills.

I invite you to consider applying this framework to some ethical dilemmas to test your thinking. This might also be an excellent exercise with your supervisor and other therapy colleagues.

Ethical decision-making in action

To help you practise ethical decision-making, read the following scenarios and consider the reflective questions.

The meeting

You attend a community event. It's a busy meeting in a room where you're expected to be for the next few hours. (It could be a workshop, political discussion group or community event about a crucial local matter.)

You arrive a bit late, the room is crowded and only a few chairs remain. One seat is next to a client who sees you enter and beckons to you, pointing out the space next to them.

In your last session, your client told you they had a sex dream about you.

Reflective questions

- What is your first emotional reaction to this? What informs that?
- How might you pay attention to your facial expression and body language?
- What might be your fears and anxieties if you accept the invitation and the possible unconscious communication?

- If they hadn't told you of the sex dream, might you behave differently?
- How might you sitting elsewhere play out in the therapy room at your next session?
- How would the purpose of the meeting affect your decision-making? Sitting in a talk where you're informed of things might be quite different to an experiential workshop or discussion group.
- If time wasn't an issue and you didn't need to respond immediately, what might you learn from invoking your inner supervisor? What questions or considerations would your supervisor be asking you?

Points to consider

Some therapists might feel uncomfortable sitting with the client for fear of stoking the erotic feelings in the client, and they are unsure they could handle them. Other therapists might feel it conveys a powerful rejection of the client's honesty and that by sitting next to the client, you are demonstrating you accept them and their erotic feelings and you know you won't be acting on them.

Yet others might say it's too distracting to sit with the client. They would take one of the few remaining seats elsewhere and work through the consequences of this potential rejection in the consulting room.

The affair

You are four sessions into a course of therapy with Alex, whose main presenting problem is their unmanageable jealousy at their partner Chris's infidelity.

You realise in the fourth session that you had a brief sexual relationship with Alex's partner six months earlier, from some unambiguous biographical data about them.

Reflective questions

- How might your thoughts and feelings at this discovery impact your ability to remain calm and focused on the client for the remainder of this session?
- Would you feel comfortable continuing with the client, or would it be better to refer them to a colleague? Would you tell them why?
- What might the consequences be of coming clean and disclosing your connection to your client's partner?
- What might be the consequences of the client discovering this via their partner?
- How might therapists from different modalities respond to this situation?
- How does your immediate felt sense align with the ethical principles outlined previously? i.e. what you want to do vs what you should do.
- If you're in a monogamous relationship, how might you judge this therapist's behaviour and boundaries? Schadenfreude?

Points to consider

If you continue with this client and they find out your affair was during the time they'd been a client, their sense of betrayal is likely compounded, and you will be implicated in it. This is likely to result in a significant therapeutic rupture. If you are a COSRT member, the client might bring a complaint against you for a breach of the Code of Ethics.

If your affair pre-dates the work, there could still be a therapeutic rupture if they discover this (from their partner).

If you declare a conflict of interest or 'personal 'reasons' which can't be disclosed, and that you need to refer to a colleague, you are likely to incur their wrath and pressure to reveal why.

If you did reveal why you need to refer, i.e. that you had slept with their partner, and their jealousy is out of control – you could be putting the life of their partner at risk.

Would you brief the therapist you're referring the client to about the full reason for the referral? Doing this puts them in an invidious position with the client, who might arrive angry and pressure them to know why you 'rejected' them.

You've got a match!

You are online dating and are withholding your own face pic. You get a message from someone whose profile also doesn't have a face pic, but the profile text is a perfect match for what you're looking for, and the profile pic is an incredibly hot body.

In their first message, they send you a face pic and a series of sexually explicit pics, and you recognise a current client.

Reflective questions

- How might this account inform your online presence/behaviour after reading this example?
- Are there any lessons from this example that you might choose to adopt or refine for your presence online?

Points to consider

Assuming that you're both on Grindr and this person hasn't seen a face pic of you, then on recognising your client from their message, this seems to be an occasion for using the 'block' button, so both of you will disappear from each other's screens. Whilst this action might cause them distress from being rejected, it could be highly awkward and shaming to send a message informing them that they are your client!

If you had been showing your face pic on your Grindr profile (as half our respondents on the survey mentioned earlier did (Davies et al., 2016), and you get cruised by a client sending you explicit pics, then perhaps one course of action would be to suggest you both talk about this at your next session. You might want to make it clear that your personal and professional boundaries prohibit any sexual contact with clients and advise them that you should both mutually block each other on the app so that you don't accidentally message each other in future.

The house party

You arrive at a house party with your partner and friends that you heard about at your local pub. It's been a tough week, and you're reasonably merry. Some other guests at the party let you in, and you get drinks in the kitchen and start talking to the other people there. After 30 minutes, the person whose party it is comes into the room, and you realise it is your ex-client.

Reflective questions

- In your opinion, is this a boundary-crossing or a boundary violation?
- Might there be circumstances in which you would remain at the party?
- If your ex-client was happy to see you and asked you to stay, how might you maintain their confidentiality if they choose to share aspects of your sessions/ relationship with their friends? How can you be sure they aren't just being polite?

Points to consider

In realising whose house you are in, it would be essential to seek a quiet moment with your former client. You would seek to reassure them that you had no idea whose house party you were visiting and offer to leave immediately. You might ask how they feel about seeing you in their space. If the therapy ended warmly and well, they might be delightfully surprised that you're there and happy for you to stay. You could be introduced to their friends and partner as the former therapist, which presents further dilemmas for you in maintaining confidentiality whilst intoxicated.

If, however, the therapy ended poorly, you would probably wish to make your apologies to the host and explain to your friends that you have a headache and are going to return home.

You might, in any event, consider raising this with your supervisor and perhaps email a further apology and explanation with an offer to discuss how they felt at your unprompted arrival.

The changing room

You're at your local gym or swimming pool with a friend, partner or children and are walking back to the lockers after your shower. You enter the communal changing room and begin to get changed when one of your current clients enters the room and starts to get undressed. They don't appear to have noticed you yet! Your companion(s) seem in a particularly chatty mood with you and are slow to get changed.

Reflective questions

- How might you feel about a client seeing you naked?
- Might you feel more comfortable with some clients than others?
- Would you have felt differently had you seen them whilst doing your workout/ swim?

Points to consider

Within the gay male community, in large towns and cities, it's common to find significant numbers of gay men being members of the same gym. If therapists were to join such a gym, they are inevitably likely to see clients there.

Britons, in general, often have an awkwardness and shame about nudity, so this answer might be subjectively different to perhaps a Nordic response, where nudity is viewed differently.

So, in essence, a British therapist would more likely seek out a private changing room and, if none were available, change quickly and quietly, using their towel to protect their modesty. If the client noticed you, it would be important to give a friendly acknowledgement if appropriate, and within the agreement you had regarding seeing each other outside of the consulting room, and leave the changing room as soon as possible.

I love you and you and you

You are in a Polycule with three others. It comprises you and your nesting partner of a decade, plus another couple whom you've been seeing separately and together for the past year. One of the other pair tells you that they've recently started dating someone new, who, unbeknown to them, is an ongoing client of yours.

Reflective questions

- What are the likely emotions you might feel here?
- How would you deal with all the emotions this raises in you?
- How would your ethical code advise you to deal with this?
- Does your own professional boundary statement cover scenarios like this or does it need updating?

Points to consider

Whilst your partners are likely to know what you do for work, you must protect your client's confidentiality and so can't be too explicit with them, assuming you learn of the client's involvement from your partner.

It would probably be best to let your client know they are dating someone in your inner circle, creating a conflicting relationship. In respecting their autonomy, offer them the choice of either finding a new therapist if they wish to pursue their new relationship or stop seeing your partner.

If your client did decide to end therapy with you, you might still want to consider ending your relationship with your polyamorous partner. Indeed, there is also the possibility that both your partner and client might decide to end with you.

If your client chooses to continue therapy with you, you may need to work on any frustration, resentment, and envy that the client carries in giving up their new relationship.

Hanging around

You are involved in your local kink community. You enjoy being tied up and suspended above the ground, floating in the air. One of your close friends is an expert in Shibari bondage (the Japanese art of intricate and beautiful rope bondage). They've asked you to be part of a demonstration they're giving at a dungeon party where it's possible clients might be present. You would be dressed only in underwear. What might be the issues for you in considering this invitation?

Reflective questions

- What's your first reaction to your friend's offer?
- Are you torn between the 'wanting' and the 'should'?
- Do you experience any conflict between professional obligations and personal autonomy?
- How would you resolve your resentment if it arises?

Points to consider

Do you feel body confident?

One of the key considerations here is perhaps asking yourself: how might you feel if a client of yours watched you as you got tied up in your underwear?

Would you feel more comfortable if you were tied up clothed? Would this be acceptable to your friend for the demo?

Are you breaking any ethical codes?

Some people might argue that such participation brings the profession into disrepute because of the connection to BDSM. How would you respond to this accusation?

Others might say you have a right to private life and that you're wearing as much as you might be if someone saw you on the beach.

Would you feel differently if your friend needed someone to receive a flogging/spanking?

Would you feel comfortable giving the flogging/spanking rather than receiving it?

Date night

It is date night, and your partner is taking you out for a romantic dinner. The restaurant is very popular and therefore reasonably crowded. You've settled into the meal and have had your first course when the maître d' escorts a couple to the only remaining spare table next to you. One of the couples is a current client who has been presenting their infidelity.

Reflective questions

- How are you feeling about the intrusion into your date night?
- How does their presence affect your conversation and rapport with your partner?
- How do you respond when the client says Hello?
- What happens if they don't acknowledge you?
- What is the impact on your perception of the client from having seen them with their partner?
- It's not clear in the example if the client is with their partner or their lover. How might you feel if they start sniping at each other, or if they become overtly flirtatious?

Points to consider

Some therapists have a non-verbal signal with their partner that they're in the vicinity of a client and may behave out of character (by becoming quieter or needing to leave). Do you have such a system in place?

In this situation, it would be very difficult to abort your meal, but their presence is likely to make a significant impact on your romantic date. It's one of those situations where you probably have to tough it out and be aware of their presence.

At the gym/pool

You're showering off after a particularly vigorous swim/workout when a client walks into the communal showers and strips off to shower. There is a reciprocal but unexpressed attraction between you two.

Reflective questions

- What do you do?
- How do you manage this additional information about your client's body?
- Do you initiate a discussion of this when you next meet or wait to see if your client brings it up?
- How might this impact the erotic feelings you have for each other?

Points to consider

Most therapists would avoid sharing that they find a client attractive as that is likely to derail the therapeutic process. However, you have both seen each other naked, which is likely to impact the work and will require some close attention in supervision.

Conclusion

By engaging with these case studies and applying the ethical decision-making frameworks outlined, I hope you will be more confident when encountering similar or entirely different real-life scenarios. You must have a clinical supervisor who is experienced and knowledgeable in the GSRD communities you are a part of. You need someone with whom you can be open and share your dilemmas and feelings without fear of embarrassment or shame. You owe this to yourself, your colleagues and, most importantly, your clients. Your supervisor needs to help you remain accountable and have the capacity to help you manage complex ethical decisions.

References

British Association for Counselling and Psychotherapy. (2018). *Ethical Framework for the Counselling Professions*. Retrieved September 5, 2022, from www.bacp.co.uk/media/3103/bacp-ethical-framework-for-the-counselling-professions-2018.pdf/

College of Sex and Relationship Therapists. (2022). *Good Therapy Code of Ethics and Practice*. Retrieved September 5, 2022, from www.cosrt.org.uk/wp-content/uploads/2022/02/COSRT-Code-of-Ethics-and-Practice-2022.pdf

Danzer, G. (2019). *Therapist Self-Disclosure*. London: Routledge.

Davies, D., & Aykroyd, M. (2002). Sexual orientation and psychological contact. In G. Wyatt & P. Sanders (Eds.), *Rogers' Therapeutic Conditions: Evolution, Theory and Practice. Volume 4: Contact and Psychological Contact Perception* (pp. 221–233). Ross-on-Wye: PCCS Books.

Davies, D., Chislett, L., Stuart, D., Palmer, R., & Sergeant, T. (2016). *The Lust Which Dare Not Speak Its Name: A Survey About App Use Among Gay and Bi Male Therapists and Sexual Health Staff*. Pink Therapy Conference Presentation, March 2016. Retrieved from https://youtu.be/1eDHec85eQs

Davies, D., & Neves, S. (2023). Gender, sex and relationship diversity therapy. In T. Hanley & L. Winter (Eds.), *The SAGE Handbook of Counselling and Psychotherapy* (5th ed.). London: Sage.

Drescher, J. (1998). *Psychoanalytic Therapy and the Gay Man*. New York: Analytic Press.

Forester-Miller, H., & Davis, T. E. (2016). *Practitioner's Guide to Ethical Decision Making* (Rev. ed.). Retrieved December 20, 2022, from https://www.counseling.org/docs/default-source/ethics/practioner-39-s-guide-to-ethical-decision-making.pdf?sfvrsn=f9e5482c_12

Freud, S. (1912). *Recommendations to Physicians Practicing Psycho-Analysis* (Standard ed., Vol. 12, pp. 109–120). London: Hogarth Press, 1958.

Gabriel, L. (2005). *Speaking the Unspeakable – The Ethics of Dual Relationships in Counselling and Psychotherapy*. London: Routledge.

Gabriel, L., & Davies, D. (2000). The management of ethical dilemmas associated with dual relationships. In C. Neal & D. Davies (Eds.), *Issues in Therapy with Lesbian, Gay, Bisexual and Transgender Clients*. Buckingham: Open University Press/McGraw Hill.

Harris, A. J. L. (2015). *To Disclose or Not to Disclose? The LGBT Therapist's Question*. DClinPsy thesis, University of Lincoln.

Jeffery, M. K., & Tweed, A. E. (2015). Clinician self-disclosure or clinician self-concealment? Lesbian, gay and bisexual mental health practitioners' experiences of disclosure in therapeutic relationships. *Counselling and Psychotherapy Research*, 15(1), 41–49. http://doi.org/10.1002/capr.12011

Lazarus, A. A., & Zur, O. (Eds.). (2002). *Dual Relationships in Psychotherapy*. New York: Springer Publishing Co.

Meyer, I. H. (2015). Resilience in the study of minority stress and health of sexual and gender minorities. *Psychology of Sexual Orientation and Gender Diversity*, 2(3), 209–213.

Pachankis, J. E., Clark, K. A., Burton, C. L., Hughto, J. M. W., Bränström, R., & Keene, D. E. (2020). Sex, status, competition, and exclusion: Intraminority stress from within the gay community and gay and bisexual men's mental health. *Journal of Personality and Social Psychology*, 119(3), 713–740. https://doi.org/10.1037/pspp0000282

Pope, K. S., Sonne, J. L., & Holroyd, J. (2005). *Sexual Feelings in Psychotherapy: Explorations for Therapists and Therapists-In-Training*. Washington, DC: American Psychological Association.

Pope, K. S., & Vasquez, M. J. T. (2016). *Ethics in Psychotherapy and Counseling: A Practical Guide* (5th ed.). London: Wiley.

Satterly, B. A. (2006). Therapist self-disclosure from a gay male perspective. *Families in Society*, 87(2), 240–247. http://doi.org/10.1606/1044-3894.3517

Shlien, J. M. (1984). *A Countertheory of Transference*. Retrieved September 15, 2021, from https://adpca.org/wp-content/uploads/2020/11/A-Counter-Theory-of-Transference_John-M.-Shlien_1.pdf

Stuart, D. (2016). Chemsex Crucible: The context and the controversy. *Journal of Family Planning and Reproductive Health Care*, 42, 295–296.

Stubbe, D. (2020). Practicing cultural competence and cultural humility in the care of diverse patients. *Focus*, 18(1), 49–51.

Tervalon, M., & Murray-Garcia, J. (1998). Cultural humility versus cultural competence: A critical distinction in defining physician training outcomes in multicultural education. *Journal of Health Care for the Poor and Underserved*, 9(2), 117–125. https://doi.org/10.1353/hpu.2010.0233

UKCP Code of Ethics and Professional Practice. (2019). Retrieved September 5, 2022, www.psychotherapy.org.uk/media/v11peyoh/ukcp-code-of-ethics-and-professional-practice-2019.pdf

Zur, O. (2022). Dual Relationships, Multiple Relationships, Boundaries, Boundary Crossings & Boundary Violations in Psychotherapy, Counseling Mental Health. Retrieved September 5, 2022, from www.zurinstitute.com/boundaries-dual-relationships/#boundaries

Conclusion

Silva Neves and Dominic Davies

The Pink Therapy series has always been about frequently bringing to the table what the heteronormative and mononormative psychotherapy trainings ignore. This book is no different. Having read this volume, we hope readers can reflect on their practice and identify the previously unseen heteronormativity and mononormativity that are so engrained (and therefore often unexamined) in how we are taught to conduct relationship therapy. It is imperative for GSRD therapists and all therapists working with relationships to pause and think about the pervasive monogamism in psychotherapy. We've explored how to work with dyads who want to open their relationships and work expertly with consensual non-monogamous relationships.

Our profession also needs to understand better marginalised populations that are often pathologised or dismissed, such as sex workers, Queer people living with chronic health issues, gay men living with HIV, and how to work ethically with each other in these populations' relationships.

Another aspect of relationships is the one with ourselves and our identities. The Trans Compass offers a unique framework for understanding the lived experience of trans people's relationships with their identities.

In this book, you have read about the critical considerations we need to have for safely and ethically working with Bi+ clients, another section of the LGBTQIA+ population that is often erased, and Queer people facing intimate partner violence, a population who requires specialist knowledge.

This book also addresses the importance of challenging our Westernised thinking in helping Queer clients with the relationship with their faith or those from non-Western identities such as African diasporan people. These gift us with the opportunity to re-think how we can support the therapeutic processes of our clients, from one-to-one intellectual conversations in a consulting room to multiple dimensions of connectedness.

Of course, we therapists need to consider our relationship with ourselves. We need to learn to develop our careers in becoming GSRD-affirmative supervisors to support our therapist community, and we need to have more honest conversations about being humans and our rights to fulfilling sex and relationships when living in the same communities as our clients.

DOI: 10.4324/9781003260561-15

As you can see, this book doesn't leave any stones unturned on the subject of Queer relationships. We are grateful to all the authors who generously contributed to the chapters of this book. Our relationship with each other, the exciting, inquisitive and nurturing professional network of Pink Therapy, is a place of 'home' and belonging for us.

Each of these valuable chapters is an introduction to frequently unexplored territory, and each topic deserves at least a whole book of its own. We look forward to seeing this evolving field grow and develop in theoretical and clinical complexity that reflects our relational worlds' complex and multifaceted nature.

If you haven't had a chance to read the companion book *Erotically Queer* yet, we're sure you will find it compelling!

If you have read our companion book, we extend our immense gratitude for your interest and commitment to serving your GSRD clients better.

Silva and Dominic

Index

9781032197241